I've G~~ot What?~~
Not Me, I'm a Man!

By John Bovaird
Houston, Tx 77082

09--25-2019

Dedication

This book is dedicated to those who've failed to realize men, too, can get breast cancer. Yeah, that's right, even you, macho man, like me; you can get it!

Along the way prior to this incident, two medical professionals deserve recognition. Special thanks to Dr. Gerald Gudarian and Dr. Luciano Gaigher for their sound advice and insight freely shared through the years. They helped me realize that to make healthier/wiser lifestyle choices, I had to listen and take heed to what they offered. .

Following my diagnosis, I give thanks to my oncologist, Dr. Craig Kovitz, for his helpful, personable, and candid conversations during the early stages of my treatment before he left MDAnderson (MDA) in 2013. We developed an extraordinary association based on trust and confidentiality. I genuinely appreciated his openness especially when I knew very little about my chances of survival and recovery.

And, lastly, to all men who have needed to be aware of their breast cancer susceptibility, this book is dedicated. It may be your chance to avoid male breast cancer (MBC), altogether, or catch the disease early.

Foreword

Although the author is in his 80s, he is still very active and fit due to a healthy lifestyle that he's followed since he was 15 years old. If you read his first book, "*Fit After 40 - Staying Fit & Healthy for the Aging Man*", you'd get a pretty good idea about who he is and how he's lived his life.

Despite all his care, however, unplanned things do happen--John developed male breast cancer (MBC). This book is about how he managed to overcome this dreaded disease. His premise is simple and uncomplicated; he wishes to reach out to those men who insist on believing (as he once did) that breast cancer will not happen to them. After all, he's a man!

There's an abundance of published/online information more accessible for women than men. Even statistics about this disease are skewed toward women. According to the American Cancer Society, breast cancer is about 100 times more common in Caucasian women than Caucasian men and 70 times more common in Afro women than Afro men. Therefore, many people don't realize men have breast tissue and are susceptible to acquiring a male version of breast cancer; uncontrolled growth of male breast tissue can develop tumors felt on exam and/or seen on imaging studies. These tumors can then spread to surrounding or distant tissues in the body with potentially lethal consequences. The American Cancer Society estimated that 2,550 new cases of invasive breast cancer would be diagnosed in the United States in 2018 with 480 men dying from the disease. Furthermore, the lifetime risk of MBC is 1 in 833 (https://www.cancer.org/cancer/breast-cancer-in-men/about/what-is-breast-cancer-in-men.html).

Through the years, the author has had discussions with other men in his life: relatives, friends, sports medicine professionals, fitness trainers, general practitioners, disease-specific medical professionals, one college professor, other aging athletes as well as lay people throughout the country before he considered writing such a book. Furthermore, he's discussed his intention to write a book about his cancer experience with women. Everyone has agreed his approach has been needed for the sake of male awareness.

Although breast cancer information has been well publicized throughout the years, it almost always is for women. For instance a recent Google© search using "Breast Cancer CDC" (https://www.cdc.gov/cancer/breast/index.htm) found a significant amount of breast cancer information (22,800,000 hits), but mostly for women whereas only a limited amount for men.

It's evident that men need to know what they can potentially go through after a MBC diagnosis, whether they'll survive the disease or treatment, and what implications they may face should breast cancer be denied. Mr. Bovaird's hope is that through more awareness, there will be heightened emphasis and research strictly focused on a cure for men.

Gerard L. Guderian, MD, MPH, MBA

Background

My primary profession is completely unrelated to medicine. Although, I wanted to become a doctor in my growing years, I decided against it for several reasons. It was going to cost a good deal of money my single mother did not have; it was going to take a long time to reach residency; and interns get little sleep. I never felt good about sleep deprivation, so, I nixed the idea. Nevertheless, I maintained my interest in the human body and what I could learn about it. In spite of my limited knowledge in this field,

In actuality, I've three professions. First and foremost, I'm a multi-certified technology audit-risk management-cybersecurity specialist with over 50 years of business experience. I'm better known as an IT audit/risk management/Cyber-security consultant. I've had my practice since 2004 and still going strong. I'm also a proud member of InfraGard affiliated with the FBI established to ensure the protection and safety of our country's infrastructure from domestic/foreign terrorism.

That said, I've, also, over 60 years' experience as a trainer giving training advice and fitness presentations. Part of that time, I've trained or coached athletes and non-athletes alike. The age range is quite broad: Boys ranging in age from 12 and 13 years old to high schoolers. Then, there've been college athletes. I've been fortunate to have trained one US Olympic sprinter in his preparation to become a professional football wide receiver.

In more recent times, I'd become multi-certified as a fitness trainer focusing on strength and conditioning.

Lastly, since I enjoy giving advice, I'd become an established author.

As a point of interest, I'm proud to have been a six year obligor in the United States Marine Corps.

What's more in years past, I competed in three iron sports beginning in my teens until my early 50s. I was nationally ranked in Olympic weightlifting, power-lifting, and bodybuilding a total of nine times. After which, I promised I'd continue to take good care of myself utilizing resistance exercise and aerobic work to maintain my health.

To this day, I train 5-6 days of each week, aerobically and anaerobically, to stay fit. I can be seen in the gym utilizing high intensity resistance exercise or running intervals on the bike/treadmill. It's been my lifestyle for years.

Why so much detail before you reach the main body of this book? I wanted to ensure you I was far from a typical senior citizen leading a sedentary life. Not only did I have an interest in health and the human body, I've effectively applied to myself what I've learned through the years. Additionally, my first book is an advice book for men 40 and older while this one deals with my cancer experience and what advice I can offer to men who are struggling with what they need to know about male breast cancer and how to minimize the risks associated with cancer recurrence.

Table of Contents

CHAPTER
I
Family

General

Whether my personal history is of any significance or has a bearing on my male breast cancer (MBC) experience, I haven't a clue. What I do know is I was forced to deal with a significant amount of stress/anxiety at a very young age until I learned there were healthier ways to cope with life. Moreover, research has indicated that to minimize risks associated with disease, stress/anxiety must be effectively managed.

Life is unpredictable when things have a way of changing, planned or not, like it or don't! Was this growth in my chest cancer or just another lump like I had when I was a teenager? What added to the mystery was I was ignorant and, simply put, I didn't know how age can change matters! Although my PCP advised me to get it removed right away, his instruction was inaptly ignored! Life's full of choices. What might be the consequence of this one?

Maybe, one domain to examine is my family tree or, perhaps, the answer can be found in my developmental years. Getting acquainted with events that transpired through adulthood could hold the solution. Most of my not so pleasant experiences became lessons in life. Let's find out what I learned, together.

It's Relative

By today's standard, both sides of my family were large. My mother had two sisters and three brothers. My father's side yielded two aunts who became nuns, two uncles, and one non-degreed white collar aunt. I lost one paternal uncle who was shot down over Germany during WWII. My dad worked in bars or restaurants most of his life. He was a remarkable cook, a talent that personally benefitted me; the way he prepared food at his home was outstandingly delicious

Economically speaking, my maternal relatives didn't fare well, except for one aunt. All were under-educated blue collar; nobody completed high school. My mom dropped out her sophomore year and worked most her life as a waitress until retirement at 65. In fact, I have the distinction of being the first on her side of the family to have graduated from high school. Although she stopped smoking and drinking somewhere in her late 50s, these bad habits took a toll on her health later in life.

As time passed on, so did my family. My maternal grandmother died in her early 60s of gangrene brought on by diabetes. One aunt died of lung cancer while the other of unknown causes precipitated by diabetes: both were in their early 60s. One uncle died of throat cancer; another died of prostate cancer.

When they passed away, they were both in their 50s. My last and oldest uncle died somewhere in his 70s of unknown causes. As a recluse who kept to himself, it was anyone's guess what caused his death. My grandfather lived the longest; he died at 99 years of age of unknown causes.

My mother's second marriage yielded a half-sister, Diane, who dropped out of school, and, finally, got a GED sometime in her 20s. There was always conflict between us because she was the favored child and, predictably, became a dependent adult. Our mother was overly-protective of her which widened the gap between us. Our values were markedly different; I was quite independent and self-reliant while Diane was the converse. We went our separate ways after I grew up and left home. I didn't stay in contact with her; it was always through her grown children or ex-husband. She got into smoking, alcohol, and drugs, not my life style at all! The tragedy in her life was Diane contracted pancreatic and uterine cancer that killed her at age 49.

Besides my maternal grandfather, my mother did remarkably well, longevity-wise. She beat colon cancer in her 70s, but remember she quit smoking and drinking? Although a good choice, those nasty habits prematurely aged her lungs, bladder, and liver. All three cancers killed her a few months away from her 90th birthday.

When my dad got out of the service sometime in the late 40s, he settled in Colorado Springs, Colorado. I met him when I was 14 years old after he moved back to Rochester, New York. He wanted more from me than what life had given him, "I've been a cook, bartender, and baker all my life. Go to college and make something of yourself!" It was good advice and validation. I regret that I never thanked him for his encouraging words before he died in 1979 at 59. He, too, was a smoker and drinker. He met his death during exploratory surgery following complaints of pain in his hip; it was cancer. He never survived the anesthesia; his liver was so badly diseased.

My father's parents, my paternal grandparents lived very close to me when I was in my teens. When my sister and I started to live with our mother, we happened to move about two blocks away by coincidence. Although, they were considered blue collar, they lived in and owned their own house. This was an uncommon occurrence amongst my extended family. Except for my maternal grandparents and one uncle in California, nobody else owned a home on my mom's side of the family. My two maternal uncles owned mobile homes while my aunts rented apartments.

Although, I don't know how old my paternal grandmother was when she transitioned, my paternal grandfather lived the longest of everyone in my family at 101 years of age.

I knew my mother's side of the family better since I lived with her when I was not in foster care. There was constant worry about money, paying bills, and whether debt would become unmanageable. It was hard, too, because most of my developmental years, my mother was a single parent. She was married to a different man other than my father when I was born, divorced this man and remarried several years later. A half-sister resulted. Then, after several volatile years, she divorced, again. It took five marriages for my mother to realize she could not successfully live with a man. It seems it was a fling since my father and her never married.

There were so many men in and out of my mother's life including boyfriends. They could all have had an effect on me; some tried to be my "friend" while others kept an emotional distance. Sometimes, I'd even get a pat on the head. With my foster care experience, I learned to accept what was or wasn't offered. Besides, I reasoned, my mother would, soon, tire of them. They were all going to temporary, anyways, so why worry about it?

There was one exception, Andy Anderson, a live-in boyfriend. Diane and I were still in foster care at the time and visited our mom on weekends. Mom was head over heels in love; this was the man. He took a sincere interest in me; it felt good. He'd even intervene when my mother attempted to grab me by the hair, beat my head against the wall, and punch me. I was 12 and in the Boy Scouts. Andy joined our troop as an assistant scout master. I was thrilled to have someone on my side at home when my sister and I visited on weekends. Well, as could have been predicted, Andy had enough and left her. She was devastated for about three years. .

To make a point, my mother ruled; she was the undisputed "boss". I was afraid for my safety if I ever asked her a question for fear it would provoke an episode of rage when I'd get literally beat up for asking. Thus, recognizing how easy it was to set her off, I never questioned why I wasn't living somewhere else within our extended family unit instead of the many foster homes.

My father was also married several times. In fact, he liked much younger women when I knew him. I met his last wife when in my mid-teens. While he was in his 30s; she appeared to be somewhere in her 20s. What I found extraordinary was she shined his shoes for him and appeared to take orders with regularity. He sure seemed "bossy" and Anne quietly complied. I wondered how long she'd put up with him.

The rest of my paternal side died of natural causes including my one aunt. She survived breast cancer in the 1960s while in her early 40s and reached old age, exactly where, I don't know. I never paid much attention to the matter or when she died. I was struggling with my own personal issues stemming from earlier life experiences. Besides, I reasoned, "I'm a man and men don't get breast cancer!"

Nevertheless, it made me think about my mortality and life shortly after I learned of her dilemma. I was in my early 20s. Outside that one instance, I felt the rest of my relatives were doing exceptionally well, health-wise.

As I reflect back on both sides of my family, I can easily see their lives were shortened due to a weakened immune system brought on by poor lifestyle choices and age. The two exceptions were my grandfathers who reached the century mark with little to no appreciable intent to make it that far. My maternal grandfather walked nearly everywhere and drank enough wine years earlier to benefit by the resveratrol. I have no idea how my other grandfather reached 101.

Just Me
"Extraordinary" actually began at birth which in part may explain how I've effectively learned to process matters differently than most. My story gets a bit bumpy at times; nonetheless, matters transparent to most people significantly impacted me.

A pre-World War II baby; it happened June, 1939 in Rochester, New York at St. Mary's Hospital. It was Flag Day, the 14th. I was about a month ahead of full term, sometime in late July. As most preemies, I was tiny weighing a scant 4lbs 4ozs. My mother was married at the time, except my father wasn't her husband. Thus, I was an out of wedlock child, born close to death as I was taken from my mother. It became my first daunting, traumatic experience on Earth. I wasn't breathing on my own.

I remember an extremely unbearable pain in the left side of my chest while a smothering sensation overwhelmed me at the same time; I couldn't breathe as hard as my frail body stubbornly tried to take in that first breath of life, it wouldn't come. The harder I tried to draw in that breath, the stronger was the chest pain. Although, my lungs doggedly insisted air could be taken in, they were denied every time. The smothering worsened until I could no longer bear my breathless existence. Finally, what physical life I had was gone; my head dropped as my body became completely limp. I surrendered and transitioned back into my spiritual state.

I could see movement in a large room below as I slowly ascended from this worldly end. There were old, large, opaque flip-glass windows with long pull cords to open and close them to my front. Downward to the right was a large white porcelain sink while just below me were big lights illuminating downward over white garbed beings focusing on another on a white table. It was too crowded to clearly see specific detail. Surely, it was the delivery room

As I continued upward into a sea of darkness, the pain subsided and the room was gone. I was floating, but something was drawing me off to my right at an angle resembling a mathematical 30 degrees. I looked ahead to see a brilliant energy form in the upper right quadrant of all this darkness. Was it possible this darkness had "corners"? At the same time, an exhilarating, wonderful, warm, serene, loving sensation that could only be described as a quality of good yet to be experienced on earth. It was all encompassing and consumed me. The strength of this amazing love and contentment could not be denied. I felt I was becoming part of it. Its power got stronger as I drew nearer, but before I was entirely devoured, another force stopped me. A nonverbal dialogue began which instructed that I had to "go back down". An ache of disappointment overwhelmed me and I reacted in kind with an "Aw, I've got to go back down?"

As the last of those silent "words" were uttered, I was whisked in a flash downward back to the delivery room. Some of the chest pain returned, but was more bearable. I could breathe; what a wonderful feeling! There was fullness in my chest for the first time! With each breathe, the pain slowly subsided. I heard voices over my crying; life had been granted!

Although, it took some doing and time, a quick-witted nurse brought my lifeless body back from the brink. My mother told me of this harrowing experience when I was ten. It placed the pain and everything else about this event into perspective for the very first time. I'll always remember how my Earthly life began outside my mother's womb.

Moving on … I'm half Italian on my mother's side with a French last name, Bovaird, but my father was Austrian-Irish. My mother argued with the courts to grant me her married name instead of his surname, McGlynn.

I have no idea when foster care started. What I can remember is I only saw my mother, intermittently, from infancy until shortly after she remarried a second time. Here's the odd part, it was never explained why I was put in foster care and why there were so many homes. I just had to go where I was taken and adjust as cruel and insensitive as it was. My feelings seemed to have never counted... At almost six years old, I was returned to my mother on a full time basis. Already, I'd been in foster care with three, possibly four different families. One particular couple wanted to adopt me when I was about two years old; my mother refused them. I never understood why and insist to this day this caring couple could have changed my life had I been given up for adoption.

Unknown to me at the time, my mother was extremely abusive and a very angry woman. Oh, I'd seen episodes every now and then: it scared me, but I was too little to be seriously impacted by them. She'd typically act out her anger or frustration on her husband or someone else. That someone else eventually became me.

As time passed, the impetus behind my mother's rage began to reveal itself. She had difficulty living and working with men. It seemed since I was growing up to resemble one of "them", I eventually became the brunt of her extreme cruelty. Her drinking and short, brutal temper spurred her anger of men including me. Tragically, these outbreaks became a way of life at home, an unhealthy one, at best. I had no recourse but to helplessly accept what my mother might do to me next. Inexplicably, however, I believed living at home was a better alternative than foster care. Perhaps, it was the brutality I interpreted as her expression of love. A sick addiction to pain taught me to accept her bizarre way of caring for me. Things could be worse. I could have no one to care for me at all.

More time had passed as I adjusted to her angry rants. Calm always followed as she tired of the pounding and yelling at me, after all, she was showing me how much she loved me. I'd quietly be still in my room; afterwards, hoping this particular episode was over. Maybe if I acted like nothing happened, there'd be peace for a while.

Husband number two and my mother were going to have a baby, except there was an unpleasant wrinkle to this blessing. Throughout most of her pregnancy, she made it abundantly clear she preferred girls over boys and hoped it was a girl. "Oh, I hope it's a girl; I hope it's a girl. Of course, you know I prefer girls!" She had to know how harmful those words were every time I heard them over and over, again. I'll always remember how much they hurt! It took me many years to recognize her insensitivity was simply another act of passive-aggression and thoughtlessness when it came to my feelings…

My sister, Diane, the much wished for girl, was born Christmas, 1945. And with her birth, sexism emerged in our household.

From the moment she arrived, Diane was getting most of the attention, now. I felt a growing resentment for simply being a boy as my baby sister took up more and more of my mother's time... There was a worsening in the way I was treated, more rejection and less attention. I wasn't loved, anymore! I wanted to believe my sister needed this close attentiveness because she was an infant. With nowhere to turn, nobody to hear me out, I had to learn to cope and accept these painful moments, silently.

As my sister grew from infancy to a very young girl, she started to get her share of verbal abuse, but was spared much of the physical violence I faced. Thus, her preferential treatment taught me just how prejudicial my mother had become.

One particular Friday evening while the three of us were waiting for my stepfather (Norman) to come home from work, I witnessed one of my mother's worst acts to date of violence. I knew it was Friday because in those days kike today, it was payday. Norman was late, dinner was getting cold. My mother took much pride in her cooking and was none too pleased with the delay. How dare Norman be late and let the food get "cold".

After what seemed a long while, we, finally, heard a rustle of keys in the hallway; the door opened. Norman, a little buzzed, carried several quart bottles of beer in a plain grocery bag to the refrigerator. Shouting ensued; I don't remember where my sister was, maybe in her playpen. I was in the kitchen with my mother by the cabinet sink. When the exchange grew heated and intense; I feared for my safety and climbed up on the cabinet sink to sit on the porcelain drain with crossed legs. Meanwhile, my mother continued her rant several feet away from Norman's face. Her back was towards me as she quickly spun around. I froze not knowing whether she was going to hit me. Instead, she flung open the cabinet drawer underneath my legs to draw out a butcher knife and swiftly whirled back to Norman. As she stepped, combatively, forward, she raised the knife in a stabbing fashion. I heard her scream," I'll kill you, you bastard!" while the open blade was plainly seen wavering in the air!

Norman fled not to return that evening. After he was gone mom threw the knife back in the open drawer never fully closing it and went to her bedroom, softly sobbing. Meanwhile, I quietly climbed down to the floor to spend the remaining tense moments in my room just off the kitchen. There was always a chance she wasn't finished with her anger and I was scared. I could never tell when an episode was entirely over. I quickly learned to be very careful.

I never saw Norman, again, and don't know when the divorce became final. Now, without an income, we grew ever so poor, struggling most of the time to make ends meet. In her humble way, my mother took housecleaning jobs about the apartment complex to make money; it kept the three of us, together.

The war had ended late the summer before and without Norman's paycheck, it got pretty bad; we had to move to Watkins Glen to live with my mother's parents. Our neighborhood there was predominantly Italian, although and oddly enough, a German family lived at the end of our street in a mobile home. All of us stayed clear of that part of the neighborhood and that family in particular. German hatred was still on everyone's mind so soon after the war.

We lived off the land (A way of life for my Italian grandparents), ate what was accessible, although, I remember we had meat rarely more than once a week. It wasn't enough to say we were close to unhealthy. I noticed, too, that most of my school friends had it better than we did; some were poorer than we were, yet, seemed to eat healthier.

As a skinny-scrawny third grader, I was easy prey for anyone who wanted to make a name for himself. I didn't know how to fight or defend myself. It played a big role with the German boys at the end of our street. After several ambushes while passing by an open field on my way home from school, I began using the other side of our street to get home even though there was no sidewalk. Those boys could easily hide in the tall weeds in that field waiting to pounce on me. I figured if they weren't on their bikes, I could out run them if I saw them, first. What they dished out was a milder version of what I got at home. Nevertheless, their beatings added to my sadness and abuse. Having been subjected to so much pain since infancy, I needed to find something that would make me feel better and happy if only for a short while.

By age eight, I got permission to go to the movies, alone, down in the Village of Watkins Glen. You could take such risks in those days without fear of being molested. There were only two theatres in town right next to each other and one of them stayed open full time. Lucky for me, this small township experienced little crime. I was safe, in spite of my mother's recklessness toward my safety. Perhaps, she was not so motivated by kindness when giving me this freedom, but my absence was an opportunity for her to be temporarily rid of me and her extra martial past.

With the mounting stress in my life, getting away was vital to my existence. Going to the movies proved a great escape full of appealing imagination. This temporary diversion worked and helped me develop strong character traits in the process. From my movie heroes like Roy Rogers, I learned to make wiser choices which only became more beneficial the older I grew.

Except, I needed to laugh more; what a wonderful feeling it was to laugh! Comedy soothed my mind and released much of my anxiety. I'd savor the antics of Abbott & Costello, Bob Hope, and others of the same genre. What a joy to get away to replace sadness with laughter. I could temporarily lose track of time, forget my despair, and escape the emotional pain. I couldn't have devised a more constructive diversion from reality had I tried!

Much to my delight, my mother frequently allowed me to go to the movies on a school night in addition to my many weekend jaunts. The *"Durango Kid"* usually played on Wednesdays. I'll never understand her reasoning for letting me attend the theatre so often, although, I sensed she didn't want me around. I must have reminded her, too often, that I was to, one day, become … a man.

Going to the movies seemed a gift, a marvelous means I had found to tolerate what I had to look forward to when I returned home. To make this euphoria last longer, I'd act out my heroes in what I'd seen on my way home or any other time in preparation for the relentless and unfounded ridicule I'd expect from my mother.

As time passed, so did the semblance of stability as I knew it. After about a year of living with my grandparents, my mother, sister, and I moved to a double family house in the valley closer to downtown where my mother worked as a soda fountain shop waitress. It was a time when sodas, milk shakes, and banana splits cost a measly 25 cents. She had no car and the walk from my grandparent's house must have been getting to her. Besides, she didn't learn to drive until some ten years later.

The owner of this house and his family lived on the other side of us. His wife was a "stay at home mom" like the neighbors across the street. They alternately cared for my sister and me while our mother worked. Both of these moms did what they could for us, but I was becoming more unmanageable. Stress was beginning to get the best of me.

Even so, I reasoned, we were living with our mother and didn't have to be in another home. This was the best part of the arrangement.

I should have been more careful of this blessing. Without warning or explanation, about 18 months, later, my sister and I were placed in foster care. We were shipped out to a neighboring town called Montour Falls about five miles away from where we lived. I had just started my instruction to be a Catholic altar boy which, regrettably, I had to give up. I never forgot that wonderful experience in the Catholic Church; I can still remember some of my Latin to this day. Nevertheless, I was too young to understand why we moved so much and wrenched away from our mother. We wouldn't see her for weeks which caused me to question whether this was all life had to offer.

For the short time we lived in that town (no more than two years), three different families cared for us. No fun; it meant adjustment to different family ways and rules every time. To better cope, my sister and I learned flexibility to survive the emotional roller coaster, physical disruption and distancing from our mother. I'd find myself lying in bed staring at the ceiling wondering and wondering why this way of life had become so commonplace for me. I could feel the ache of my mother's absence in spite of her sick, abusive love, a kind I failed to understand, but became addicted to as I grew older.

Nevertheless, my memories would drift back to a happier time with that couple who had wanted to adopt me. I'd imagine how much better it might have been instead of all this strife and unsettling life never knowing when calm would replace the agony of insecurity and never truly belonging. In the meanwhile, these instabilities created havoc in my soul. Was there anyone or anything we could trust and feel secure with?

While staying at one of these foster homes, I landed myself in serious trouble. There were times when the father wouldn't come home from work until after dark when all of us children were in bed. During the earlier part of the evening, I had time on my hands and began playing with matches in the bathroom. They were on the back of the toilet and there was plenty of toilet paper. I found the temptation too hard to resist. I'd act out something I cannot remember, today, and watch the flames shoot from the toilet.

One night, they shot up too far and fast; I put the toilet seat down quickly to smother the flames and quietly to not be heard. Except, I burned the underside. The smoldering gave off a strong odor as I examined the badly scorched seat. Some of the smoke drifted into the other room where the foster mother picked up the scent and heard the commotion in the bathroom. I knew I was in trouble. After her scolding, I was sent to bed to wait for the father's return home

When he arrived, I was still awake worrying about what he'd do to me. I acted asleep when he came to my bedroom area, a larger room partitioned by shower curtains. As the sound of the curtains screeched open, he briskly wrenched down my pajama bottoms. I could hear the anger in his breathing as he relentlessly continued beating me and beating me with his hand until he ran out of breath. He was panting and wheezing for air when he finally stopped. I don't remember when I fell asleep or for how long. I do know my rear end was badly bruised for days. I never told anyone nor did I ever play with fire, again.

By summer of 1950, I had just turned eleven. The three of us were, together, back in Rochester, New York which meant more foster care and separation from our mother. My heart sank when I learned we'd be in another home. Despite being in the same city, we had to look forward to the same unsettling routine all over, again, but with a different family. It'll be the familiar coldness, distance with some of the same as well as different rules.

There was a "blessing" for us this time around. Our mother would pick us up early Friday evenings every weekend and return us that Sunday by 7pm. This type of arrangement was a first for us. Boy, did we ever look forward to Fridays! In spite of the abuse from our mother and the emotional distance endured in foster care, weekends were worth our excitement! Tragically, the return to foster care on Sundays was quite painful...

This particular home was unlike the rest we'd ever lived in. Instead of a house in the suburbs, it was an apartment on the second floor in a building in downtown Rochester. I could see a car dealership across the street and beside us was a baby shoe factory. Behind us sat a body shop and used car lots with a large billboard advertising the latest movie attractions in town.

Another blessing for us was a single parent-mother in her 30s ran this home, another first. When my sister and I were introduced, I sensed right away this woman wasn't that thrilled about taking us in, no warmth or friendliness radiated just a meek, insincere "Hello". I could see the dread in her eyes, but, I guessed, the money my mother was to pay her would be worth her struggle. This go-around, we had "company": a daughter of the foster mother about ten years old and another foster child, a boy, who looked to be about eight. At least, there was no father to have to put up with this time.

Even though, I shared a bedroom with this boy; we never had much to talk about or share. Thus, we'd, typically, keep to ourselves; besides, I didn't much care for his bitter, cynical outlook. I had enough of that crap in my own life; I didn't need to hear about his. .

Every time we were returned to the home, I'd hurt all over again. The pain and unhappiness lay forgotten over the weekend only to return on our bus ride back to foster care. There was little conversation or chatter the closer we got to the home. I remember seeing other children on the bus with their parents clambering about, laughing, seemingly happy totally unlike what my sister and I were feeling. There'd be the drudgery and sadness lasting all week long until the next Friday. Each and every time, my heart sank; I could only internalize what I felt for fear I'd be ridiculed if anyone heard me cry. There was no one to confide in; how I wished there was someone who'd listen while I talked away my unhappiness! That familiar ache would always ask "When was this way of life going to end?"

Diane and I went through three more foster homes inside the next three years before we began living with our mother full time. The three of us, together, was a first since we left Watkins Glen. I was 14 years old and Diane's built in babysitter after 7:30PN every school night. I'd get razzed by my buddies because I had to leave to care for my "little" sister. Mom usually came home from a long day of waitressing close to 9PM.

Life was quite extraordinary living in so many different homes. I didn't know who to trust nor did I feel completely secure knowing everything around me was temporary; we could pull up stakes at any time. Moreover, not knowing who could be entrusted with our deepest thoughts and fears left a deep emptiness inside me. Without a sense of inner peace, fear always loomed that we'd be taken out of one home to be rendered to another without explanation or warning. At one time, I could count up to 20 families who either cared for us while our mother worked or whom we lived with until I was a teenager. Today, I can only account for about half that many. The average time spent in foster care varied and lasted no more than 18 months or so.

With all this instability, I became conscious of socio-economics at an early age. I could see how different families struggled with debt, whether they succeeded or failed and what they did to compensate. The various outcomes taught me how to better manage my affairs, a lesson I carried with me into adulthood. Adjustment and flexibility proved a constant battle, but helped my sister and me survive the different lifestyles and rules.

Feeling "second best" in those homes was typically heartbreaking. Such feelings would most often surface when the foster-daddy came home from work; he'd get on the floor to play with all us, kids, at first. However, as the seconds ticked by, Diane and I were discarded, ignored, left on the sidelines on our knees, enviously, watching daddy play with his own. And, watch we did as he continued to laugh and play as though we didn't exist. Oh, how we both wished we'd get a few more moments of that quality time! We wanted to belong so badly, yet, knew full well that we did not. Those begrudging moments only added to my growing sadness and resentment. My anger grew, but I had no means to release or calm it.

Not all was lost; there was one significant positive in foster care, namely, the food. Until I reached the age of 12, Diane and I were fed better in foster care than at home. Our mom could only afford so much and knew little about nutrition. She thought milk was thee food and made certain we got our share, but fell short of including other better quality foods like meats, vegetables, and fruit mostly because they cost more.

However, things must have turned around for my mother. Maybe, she was making better money or maybe having a live-in boyfriend's help was the answer. Whatever it was, those weekend meals were exceptional compared to earlier years.

Unfortunately, Mom's happiness ended almost as quickly as it began when her boyfriend broke it off. I liked him; I desperately needed someone who took an active interest in me like he did. As a chronically anxious teenager trying to make sense to his life, all of this was compounded by instability, insecurity and the unsettling notion that I couldn't trust anyone. I had this belief this man could've potentially benefit me in some way, except, now, he was gone. Not only was his absence disappointing, it left my mother alone and depressed for some time. Intuitively, I distanced myself from her, again, for fear she'd act out her grief on me.

Funny how things happen … just before I was to leave the last foster home in April, 1953, my biological father called me from Colorado; he must have gotten the number from my mother. He'd settled in Colorado Springs after the War and decided to move back to Rochester to temporarily live with his parents. He sounded pleasant on the phone and sent me some gifts and mementoes from his time during the War while in the Army Air Corps. I met him the next year and noticed right away he liked beer, younger women and cigarettes!

Well, summer of '53, Diane and I started living full time with our mother. Being together for the first time after years of foster care, separation, and intermittent weekend visits made the three of us realize how little we actually knew of each other. Matters frequently got tense and brutally abusive for me when our mom was drinking. This latest breakup made her an emotional wreck! She must have really cared for this guy and felt quite lonely without him. What's more, now, she only had herself to pay the bills and care for us. With all this strife, I asked myself, "Was this the stable home life my sister and I longed for when in foster care?"

On the other hand, having been abused for so long, we accepted whatever we got as normal. Surely, living with our mother was a better alternative than anything else!

I was of high school age, now, but just as skinny and scrawny as ever. Although I was stuck home babysitting school nights, I found ways to get out on weekends. Ordinarily, mom wouldn't let me go anywhere which isolated me from school friends. Fortunately, my maternal aunt and uncle persuaded her to give me weekend time away even after dark as long as I returned before 10pm. Knowing how cruel my mother was, I made certain I was on time. Boy, did I ever look forward to weekends and freedom with my friends as long as I was home by ten!

Playing high school sports helped me find another way to get "out". There were night football games under the lights on Fridays and Saturdays. Even though I was a "bench warmer" in the beginning, being on the team meant I was allowed night game time away from home, possibly after 10PM which absolutely thrilled me!

I didn't stay on the bench for long. By my sophomore year, I became a three letter man not to be macho or popular, but, rather, playing sports was a great tension release from stress at home. There was track and wrestling besides football. I noticed, too, that I was maturing and packing on some muscle from excelling in these sports. What's more, I was getting validation from teachers, coaches, and peers for what I'd accomplished in the classroom as well as on the playing field. I got no such accolades from home, except from my aunt and uncle when they visited. I looked forward to time in school and I was learning good social skills there. Besides, it was more fun than spending idle time alone at home feeling confined, resented, unwanted, and in the way.

A wonderful man and friend, our next door neighbor encouraged me to exercise using his homemade barbell. A plumber by trade, he looked quite the part from having worked out with it. I began weight-bearing, resistance exercise at 15 and through his encouragements joined the YMCA the next year to further my athleticism. I was gaining body weight and getting stronger while setting teenage Western NY Olympic weightlifting records in AAU sanctioned meets. All this strength training helped me in my school sports.

Having turned down sex several times due to ignorance and fear, my first experience was at 16 with a girl two years older than me. There were times I'd see my father and he'd give me great advice suggesting I go out with older women in the beginning. "They'll teach you what you need to know". Walking away from that first intimate encounter caused me to question why girls were so attracted to me. Positive reinforcement given from the opposite sex was unheard of at home. I sensed one possible reason was my mother's growing resentment; she loathed what I was growing into … another man.

Did I ever get family praise, validation or reinforcement? Yes, but strictly from my aunt and uncle who encouraged me to do better in the classroom and on the playing field. They were the ones who attended most of my football games even when I "warmed the bench". It made me question whether my aunt was actually my mother; she treated me so much better. I got no such support from my mother; she never attended any of my school functions including graduation. Nobody knew the difficulty I felt achieving what I did in school without one encouraging word from home. I cannot remember a time when my mother openly expressed her pride in what I'd accomplished. A cold lesson was learned; if I was to achieve anything in life, it would be entirely up to me.

After high school graduation exercises were over, I returned home to be met with a big surprise. My aunt instructed me to wait outside while she got my mother and uncle. As the three of them approached, I saw tears sliding down my mother's cheek; I'd never seen her act this way towards me before. She had a small package in her hand. As I was approached, it took several seconds for her to recompose herself. This extraordinary display was way out of her character and had me delightfully surprised! It was hard to believe my mom was feeling this way about me! What a touching moment! With some hesitation while holding back more tears, my mother handed me the package, expressing her pride in my graduation. I silented asked why had she waited so long? That question was never to be answered!

The package? Inside laid a watch to commemorate me being the first on her side of the family to have graduated from high school. It took four generations of our Italian family to have someone graduate from high school!

Meanwhile, I'd become more serious about bodybuilding and strength competitions. I believed that to maintain my fitness after high school, resistance exercise was the direction I wanted to take. To do well, I recognized the importance of health and nutrition for athletic excellence and a wholesome lifestyle.
+++
Drinking and smoking had always been a sign of growing up to me. Eighteen was the magic drinking age in NYS at the time. My senses told me it wouldn't be something of benefit judging from what I'd seen at home. I never drank very much, didn't like the flavored alcohol although I was partial to wine, a full bodied red. I don't think I ever got wasted more than a dozen times in my entire life time. As far as tobacco went, I tried chewing it as well as smoking cigars, stogies, cigarettes, and the pipe. The smothering sensation of smoke entering my chest seemed extremely unnatural; the dryness that followed was of no help, either.

By the time I started college, I continued to compete in Olympic weightlifting and bodybuilding. For my efforts, I gained regional, state, and national rankings. In addition to training, I was also trying to juggle a full time job with college night school classes, and studying. It got tense at home with the apartment being so small. The only two places I could study were at the desk in the foyer next to the living room or at the kitchen table. My bedroom was out; there was only room for a bed and dresser. Besides, the lighting was poor for studying. My request for a desk and lamp was rejected and the distraction from the TV proved overwhelming. Mom was unwilling to turn the volume down to make studying easier. She made it very clear, "This is my place!" She paid the bills and what she would/wouldn't do was strictly up to her. Frankly, I think my mother loathed my ambition and resented that I wanted more in life than just a high school diploma. I believe it was her intent to make it just as difficult as she could for me to study so I'd fail. No surprise, I dropped out of college due to failing grades my first year.

With local newspaper coverage, my physical development, and winning/placing in local weightlifting and physique contests, my popularity with the local ladies soared. I was ignorant about their attraction, but cautiously accommodating, nonetheless. I finally figured out I could pick and choose; it was all up to me which was quite new. What a life! I, now, wish I'd paid more attention to the ladies while in high school!

I dated around to further my social skill sets, but my naivety ignored the red flags associated with unhealthy women. I was attracting the wrong kind. To add to the mess, I didn't know how to be a good boyfriend with all the emotional baggage I was carrying around.

Nevertheless, I met a not so good match and started a rocky relationship in my early 20s. By then, my hormones were in high gear! Being in a relationship was new and scary. Carol, 19, was a high school dropout who was attending a business school to obtain applicable business skill sets. Trust was an issue right away. Shortly after we met, we became intimate which to me meant we were exclusive. Clearly, it didn't mean the same to her; her hormones were raging, too! She was quite disloyal! Despite Carol's several transgressions, we got back together. Fool that I was I forgave her. She eventually got pregnant and we married. Being a father was very important to me. This child was going to have a father unlike me! We both were unprepared to settle down, nevertheless, I was determined this child would not experience what I did, never knowing what it was like to have a father!

Later, when things started dissolving, my wife and I went to marriage counselling. Carol didn't like it and refused to do her "homework", thus, it failed to improve our marriage. Much to my delight, I began to learn more about me and realized the benefit of therapy. I wanted so much to be a better man, to be better than I used to be.

In the meantime, some 13 months after our first son, we had a second boy. From what I'd seen and feedback from friends, Carol disliked domestic life and became unfaithful. We eventually separated and divorced; I was awarded full custody after it was clear, Carol became pregnant by her lover. Now, I'm a single parent with two boys. What do I do?

Wishing to avoid history repeating itself, that's exactly what happened. Sadly, after I left my wife, I reluctantly placed my boys in voluntary foster care. With my meager pay, I couldn't afford a full time sitter nor could I trust anyone to care for them while I worked, attended night classes, and trained. Their hours would have been too long and unaffordable for me. Instead, I chose foster care and depended on Social Services to effectively screen foster parents before my boys were placed in their care. In total, my sons spent about 30 months in foster care with visitations every two weeks.

In spite of the positive things going on in my life, I was unhappy, depressed, and so messed up. I wanted to try LSD. I read a good deal about what acid did and became fascinated with the notion of psychedelic trips. As it turned out I wasn't desperate enough to experience such a trip nor did I ever seek out an opportunity. Although, I was on the edge, I stayed on this side of reasonableness.

So much stress accompanied this part of my life. Besides being a father, I was a competitor and part time student while working full time. I was so glad to have a physical release for the anxiety I felt through this first decade of adulthood. I really cannot remember how I managed everything without going whacko, but somehow I did. I even passed my college courses scoring surprisingly higher than anticipated. I was serious about studying and graduating, but the going was far from easy.

Several national rankings and flings later, I was in my late 20s and remarried. Her name was Patricia, eight years younger, and some college education. I was making better choices; one of which was to stop competing to improve my chances of a lasting marriage. I bought equipment, improvised, and worked out in my basement to stay in condition. Three months after we married just before Christmas, my boys began to live with us; we were a family, again. Although, I continued to workout and earned a degree, being a good dad and husband became paramount. My wife even helped me complete my first undergraduate studies for which I'll always be grateful. Life was good; all appeared to be going smoothly.

I thought it was unfair my wife had to take birth control pills to avoid pregnancy. So, I decided it was better to get a vasectomy and became officially sterile the summer of '73. Unknown at the time, this procedure could play a significant health role later in my life.

While at Xerox, our family relocated to Texas; that proved an exciting time in all our lives. A team of us from Rochester volunteered to be a part of a new word-processing division in North Dallas. Xerox was the copier king of America at the time, but was breaking ground in the word processing business. I was a Quality Assurance engineer. Our family settled in Denton near the University of North Texas. Xerox encouraged me to get a four year degree if I wanted to get anywhere in the organization. I complied and attended night classes, but it put a strain on our marriage, Pat and me. She grew quite discontented and neglected with less quality time replaced with attending classes and studies. An emotional distance widened as I focused more on academics than her. In fact, she thought I had become unfaithful. There was no truth to that notion at all, but I could not convince her.

Five years, later, I'm about to turn 40 and separated from my second wife. Our daughter, Heather, was taken with her which deeply hurt me. Being her part time father significantly impacted our association later in life. We were no longer a family and I was crushed! I wanted that marriage so bad, except night classes and studies took away what we once had. The emotional gap between my neglected wife and me could no longer be narrowed without intervention and Pat hated counselling. With absence of commitment, my wife abandoned our family with no explanation. To worsen matters, I didn't feel right without Heather in what was left of our household. I was given the "leftovers": my teenage boys, a mortgage, and child support for our daughter.

Instead of support from my wife and partner, I got anger and resentment. Our separation was devastating to me. I missed my wife and daughter; I ached for quality time with them. Helplessness overwhelmed me until I realized I had to do something to keep my head straight. I had to survive this most heartbreaking event in my life.

Joining Parents Without Partners changed everything; I began to have the time of my life. It was dance, dance, dance, the disco era and I took lessons. I met a lot of ladies and, then, this special one, Margaret. Her timing was right; she gave me so much more than what I had in my marriage. We connected, intensely; this short-lived relationship was the best I'd had to that point in my life. But this lady was deceptive; I was used as an in-between until she could settle in California with the man she kept in contact with while simultaneously being involved with me. What we had painfully ended which shot my anxiety up; I was running scared! I'd never had anxiety attacks until now and, typically, they'd occur at my most vulnerable time when I was alone at night in bed. Eventually, they subsided as the pain of the breakup weakened over time.

During all this strife, Xerox was implementing a plan to redeploy to California and, by coincidence; all my remaining classes to graduate were offered only during the daytime. I took a great severance package which was wisely used to finish my degree. With the "leftovers", I started my master's program whose work I loved! Sadly, I had to drop out with dwindling funds and return to work.

With all my other expenses, it took creative financing and food stamps to keep my head above water as long as I did. I was proud to say I'd done it with an undergrad GPA of 3.8, solely dependent on myself!

Pat and I divorced in the interim, her doing not mine. I'll never understand why she filed after I made it abundantly clear during our separation I wanted us, our family, and marriage. Again, Pat never took the time to explain herself; she just steamrolled ahead with the notion she was the only one who counted.

Entering my 40s, I never thought of gearing up to compete, again, until one evening while watching TV, I saw an ad for a Dallas physique contest for competitors over 40 years old. I, immediately, got the bug to compete, again. I wasn't so old after all and figured I'm single, my boys are in their late teens, and I no longer have the complications of marriage.

Although, I became wiser throughout this time, I remarried out of desperation. Ellen, originally from NYC, was ten years younger than me, and she worked out. Like most rebounders, there was little good about this relationship; we separated, reconnected to separate, again and again before it, finally, ended. There was so much deception and dishonesty I was ignorant about until years later when her daughter, Hillary, told me. What a relief when we divorced. I decided marriage that late in life wasn't for me. I was still making poor choices when it came to women. I resolved therapy and self-help material would benefit me more than being with an unhealthy partner. I learned to be self-sufficient and live without anyone in my life. Therapy, also, helped me realize to attract healthy women, I had to get emotionally healthy, first.

Meanwhile on the competitive scene, a significant change had been added, the common place use of steroids. To compete and win, now, you had to use and I wanted to win. I found a doctor who prescribed a scheduled regimen of steroids for me. For a guy about 5'7", I "blew" up to a lean 185lbs. with just 3-4% body fat. It took 17 short months of hard training to achieve regional caliber and I won my division in the Mr. Over 40 Southwestern America Physique Competition. That placement automatically awarded me national ranking which qualified me for the Mr. Over 40 America where I placed in the top ten in the country, another national ranking. I used for less than three years and did quite well! I might have continued using, but the doctor, my steroid supplier, was run out of town which ended my drug use. Good thing because with extended use I may have had a permanent heart condition or died.

Work became very important during this stage of my life. I finally found a profession I genuinely enjoyed. It didn't matter whether it was called information technology audit, risk management, or compliance, they were all closely related. To demonstrate my seriousness, I obtained my first professional certification as a certified information systems auditor better known as CISA. Three more professional certs were to follow.

On the singles' scene, I met Amber, an attractive, intelligent 42 year old high school teacher. What I failed to realize was she had become my second raging alcoholic and I didn't know how to cope with the situation, let along end it. Our on-again, off-again relationship lasted for years with me unable to break it off and stay healthy without her. Much of her rage resembled what I'd experienced in my growing years. Could there be a connection?

By this point, I was closing in on 50; aerobic exercise became a significant addition to my workouts. I learned you can reduce your risk of heart stroke with a rest heart rate (RHR) under 70 bpm. My goal was to stay below that benchmark which meant my weekly intense anaerobic routine had to make room for aerobics.

After I passed the half century mark, I noticed a change in my libido. How could I get this part of aging corrected? Someone mentioned a urologist, but I put it off. Hey, I was tied up with more "important" matters. What, exactly, were they? To this day, I still, haven't a clue!

About the time I was prepping for the Over 50 Mr. USA physique competition, I finally took the time to see a urologist. His examination revealed I had hypogonadism. Simply put, my body wasn't producing enough testosterone and my testicles had reduced in size due to my steroid use some seven years prior. I was instructed to have my condition closely monitored and to begin testosterone replacement therapy (TRT) if necessary. Smart ass me, I ignored his advice figuring it was not a big deal. I'd get it resolved on my own. This hormonal imbalance continued for another 16 years. Besides, I reasoned that "little blue" pill was about to be marketed and that's all I needed to "keep" me going. I had all the answers, didn't I?

Remember Amber +the alcoholic? Due to a fine gym friend, I began an Al-Anon 12 Step program in 1991. It's similar to AA, but is for non-alcoholics influenced by someone else's drinking, although, you could, also, be an alcoholic. I was not and never have been one. There was little effect at the start because I had this notion my recovery was going to fix my alcoholic (That was a lie!). I didn't attend many meetings, consistently, until I moved to Houston for an outstanding job opportunity. Now that I was many miles away from this lady and saw her less, I became more serious about my recovery. Without her influence, I could set healthier boundaries; I learned how to say "no" and mean it. In the beginning, it was a painful awakening, but persistence and faith got me through. I finally ended this sick relationship altogether in 1998 some nine years after I'd met this woman. Many lessons learned was the price I paid.

One of them was I benefitted more from Al-Anon and therapy. Counselling revealed I had an addiction to abuse and pain. Thanks, Mom! As time passed I successfully broke away from the binding emotional ties of dependency, never to put up with abuse, again. Or would I?
.

My 60s saw me through three more unhealthy relationships, two were alcoholics while one was just plain sick with paranoia, OCD, acute mistrust, deception, and dishonesty. Noting there was nothing healthy in the relationships, I broke all of them off.

Moreover, I became estranged from my daughter, Heather, in April 2000. One of the major failures in my marriage to her mother, Pat, was the absence of open, honest communication. This very characteristic my former wife lacked was unfortunately absent from our daughter's persona. This inability to effectively communicate in combination with me disappointing her on my last visit severed all communication. I've unsuccessfully tried through the years to reach out and reconcile. Rejection has always been difficult for me. On my last attempt I got her on the phone only to be hung up on. Nevertheless, I pray for Heather every day and wonder how she explains away her choice to reject this side of her family, me, her brothers and their families! I wish she and her mother could forgive and learn to effectively communicate feelings.

Through my professional investigative work, I've learned Heather is unmarried and in partnership with a Tucker. They've owned a home in South Dallas for a number of years. Tragically, she had a miscarriage, a son,

I met a fellow Al-Anon-er, a therapist, while attending Al-Anon meetings. We became good friends. I, also, saw him as a mentor and sponsor. While I helped him with health and fitness issues, he counseled me, gratis. After I ended a relationship with my very last alcoholic, the separation proved exceedingly painful. I pleaded with my friend for guidance in response to which he gave several profound instructions that will always stay with me.

One, I possessed this quantum energy that attracted unhealthy women due to the exposure of abuse and alcoholism in my developmental years. I had to recognize and pay attention to the red flags when considering a relationship. Lastly, I'd become fully aware this sordid attraction would always be part of me for the rest of my life! My task? To attract healthy women, I had to make healthier choices.

Talk about effective application … I must have turned down over a dozen potentially unhealthy relationships by rigidly following my counselor's advice and what I'd learned from the Al-Anon Recovery Program.

However, what about the very first alcoholic in my life? Amazingly, it took until I was 65 years of age to assert what I lacked the courage to say earlier in life to my mother. She, now, knew my boundaries; I wouldn't put up with her anger or abuse, anymore. A huge emotional weight had been lifted; I could walk straighter. As a final rejection, she refused to allow me to be by her side on her death bed. With her passing, I'd never be disregarded by her, again! Moreover, I've hoped and prayed she be lifted from all her earthly pain for I've never known a more angrier or unhappy woman, here, on Earth!

At nearly 69 years of age I, finally took the time to have my testosterone (T) checked. My Primary Care Physician (PCP) recommended "T" injections every two weeks, beginning immediately. I was way below the normal range for a healthy adult male. I'd been off steroids for 23 years before I started TRT. Nobody knew of the hormonal imbalance I'd subjected myself to for one third my life. Did it make my system estrogen-estradiol dominant? No one knew because it was never a consideration or part of the blood work, although, my research says "yes".

Another decade and more went by; I'm in my early 80s now and exceedingly grateful for my Al-Anon friend's council. I've missed him since his transition in October, 2004 of lung cancer.

Conclusion
My childhood was abundantly extraordinary. Although, there were sparse times during which Diane and I lived with our mother, typically someone else cared for us. These substitute parents were the ones who heavily influenced our personal values during our developmental years. Then at 14 years of age, I became subjected to extreme verbal and physical abuse on a full time basis living in what my sister and I considered home. The atmosphere was a tense and fearful one where we never knew when a raging episode would emerge. Nevertheless, we thought the way our mother treated us was as close to "normal" as we'd ever see. What's more, I'd become addicted to the physical pain over time; it was the only attention I could depend from my mother. I recall a moment of anger when she pulled my hair and punched me against

the wall. A sick thought raced through my mind, "Oh, she loves me!" Such were the affections from my non-recovering alcoholic mother!

The challenges during my developmental years created an ever so slanted view of life and suggested what could be in store for me as an adult unless I changed. I was naïve and ill-equipped to effectively cope; I stumbled and oft times fell short of expectations. What I learned was if I was to achieve anything, it would be entirely up to me and my resourcefulness without family intervention, support, handouts, inheritances, or gratuities of any sort. I would be solely in charge of my destiny; it was the ultimate in self-reliance. Although, I became successful as an iron sport competitor, I had a ways to go before transforming into a wholesome, reasonable adult man. It took determination, time, focus, therapy, and a concerted effort to successfully get over most of my wretched past.

Memories of commonplace physical violence, resentment, rejection, and a relentless diatribe of cruel words, undeniably, were a significant part of my growing years. These wounds will indeed never be completely healed. A desire to be a better man has driven me to achieve as close to a balanced life as I've been capable.

 In spite of it all, I'll always wonder what life would have been like had I been adopted by that wonderful, loving couple. They, alone, cared for me with an unconditional love I'd experienced with no one else; I never saw it, again, ever, not even from my own mother. My tragedy is I'd only known these wonderful, would-be parents for a short time during infancy while my blessing was I'd come to know them and how genuine love felt as it was so freely shared between the three of us. I miss them …

Chapter
II
The Challenge

General

You deserve to be cautioned about the material in this book, moving forward. I've been involved with exercise in general ever since I was told how skinny I was at age eight! Resistance and aerobic exercise became a norm for me at 15. Thus, I consider the way I feel via how well I perform in the gym as my benchmark for normalcy. It may prove to be quite foreign to you. Nonetheless, you're going to find a good deal of emphasis throughout this book on how I feel by way of the gym. Mind you, it's been part of my lifestyle for a long time, bear with me!

Before I go into detail about my disease specifics, let's discuss the disease in general, first, and what might be done before you get it. The way most men think about health and annual medical checkups is they can 'fix" it, themselves. Based on that belief, consider yourself fortunate if you haven't been diagnosed with cancer. One wise choice to minimize the risks associated with disease is to obtain credible information beforehand. Age, lifestyle choices, physical condition, and genes play significant roles in health. More to consider is, how robust your immune system has become due to age and how effective you've managed disease leading to advanced age. Most importantly, choices made as you got older will determine how well you've been to avoid disease, altogether, let alone cancer.

According to AARP.org, September, 13, 2016, a national telephone survey was conducted comprised of about 500 men ages 18-70. The survey divided the results by generation: millennials (ages 18 to 35), Gen Xers (36 to 51) and baby boomers (52 to 70).

Their findings indicated men are more likely to talk to their guy buddies about current events, sports, their job or children and most anything else other than their health.

When they opened up about such matters, they'd usually discuss close calls or sports injuries while nothing was mentioned about personal or intimate health problems. Such openness typically does not happen and when men do open up, it's quite rare. Most men believe it's embarrassing to talk about their health.

To illustrate, the survey showed that 53% of men said their health wasn't something they talked about. What's more, they put off seeing their PCP for anything. Further, about 60% said they only go after a symptom or problem reached a point where they cannot tolerate it, anymore or they've been unable to "fix" it, themselves. Admittedly, some 20% say the only reason they'd see their doctor was to stop being nagged by someone close to them about their current ailment.

The purpose of the survey was, in part, to get men to pay attention to their health needs and determine whether men knew at what age they should begin preventive screenings (i.e., PSA test or colonoscopy). Unfortunately, most men had no idea when they should start these screenings.

Baby boomers were the most private about their personal health. Nearly 50% of the men in this age bracket refused to discuss health with their male friends because they ""don't feel it's any of their business."" And while 54% of the men would talk to their spouse or significant other, 26% of the men wouldn't discuss personal issues with anyone.

Millennials and Gen Xers were more open and forthcoming. Nearly half of millennials and 44% of Gen Xers said they could discuss health topics with more than one trusted individual compared with just 29% of the baby boomers.

Additional survey results suggested different priorities dependent on which age group you belong. For some reason, having children caused men to be less talkative about health issues. Men without children were most open to talking with their male friends about their health. In fact, about 52% said they've confided in friends, compared with only 36% percent of men with children.

Dependent on their health, heart attack worries slightly outranked concerns about cancer. About 44%t of men were most concerned about preventing a heart attack. In comparison 42% were worried about cancer. Interestingly, men were just as concerned about gaining weight (24%) as having a stroke (23%).

Of significance was what concerned men most about their life in the next 10 years. Baby boomer men had a tie between their health and the well-being of their family; financial stability was a distant third. For those under 50, well-being of family and financial stability were more important than their own health. I suspect the main reason why men under 50 were less concerned about their health was they believed they were healthier and didn't have health issues worthy of medical attention.

Just 35% of men across all age groups knew that age 50 was the correct age to begin testing for colon and rectal cancer with a colonoscopy. However, baby boomers were more likely to know than men under 50 about the right starting age.

The Urology Care Foundation recommends that healthy, low-risk men get a PSA test for prostate cancer starting at age 55. Conversely, on average, survey respondents across all age groups thought they should start at age 42.

Based on this study and conversations I've had with other men, most of us need to come to terms with openly discussing health concerns, sooner than later. The macho barrier of silence has to be broken to effectively diagnose and prevent cancer in men at an earlier age and diagnostic stage.

Male Breast Cancer Awareness

First and foremost, everyone needs to know breast cancer also affects men; an enormous awareness campaign should be launched. Unfortunately, most men, today, believe men cannot and do not get breast cancer. What makes this urgency significant is most everyone believes it's strictly a woman's disease. Cancer.gov says there's a lack of male awareness in the United States. What's more, the entire world needs to know the risks men face contracting this disease. For instance, October of every year is designated as Breast Cancer Awareness month. When has anyone ever heard that men can get breast cancer in any of the media ads? The answer continues to be "Never!"

Then there's the research, data, and statistics; they're all skewed towards women. Up to one percent (0.006-0.01%; 1200-2000) of all annual breast cancer cases (200,000) in the United States are male. Most studies include male statistics with female breast cancer indicators which skews the analysis regarding men. Male physiology is different than the female. Thus, there should be independent studies strictly for men, except we're in the minority. Changing current beliefs and priorities would be a challenge which brings me back to MBC awareness. It doesn't exist.

For example, I've had several not so positive experiences with the *Houston Chronicle*. A successful awareness campaign would require publicity and fund raising. Instead, public attention has focused on "thinking pink" especially in October of every year. The public is ill-informed about men acquiring this dreaded disease. My personal efforts to get this information out in the forefront has been stymied or ignored altogether.

For instance, October of 2013, I made several phone calls and left messages at the *Houston Chronicle* to publicize male breast cancer. When I got a callback, I'd hear "I'll pass it on." which got old. After I heard that same reply from the last caller, I asked, "When is "it" going to stop?" After a strained period of silence, the caller encouraged me to continue my effort to speak with someone and quickly countered with, "… although, it wasn't me!" What's more, this lady was unable to supply me with a name of someone I could speak with at the *Chronicle* while insisting I continue with what I believed to be vital information to the public. And how do I accomplish that task when no one wishes to speak with me? No answer, just silence!

After we hung up, I wondered if this lady didn't know who I could speak with. Furthermore, who was she "going to pass it on" to? It was too late; I didn't have her name or number to call back. No one else returned my calls for the remainder of October, 2013. So much for the character of those at the *Houston Chronicle*!

Similarly, I've called and written emails to the Houston Chronicle in late September, 2016. I began my trek by sending an email to "City Desk" and "Breaking News". I followed up with a call and spoke with a pleasant sounding lady; her name was Anna. She explained that Ms. Elizabeth Pudwill, the person I'd want to speak with, was out of the office. Anna seemed a good listener and sympathetic to my cause. I was provided with Ms. Pudwill's email addr and immediately wrote to her.

I waited until mid-morning of the next day to allow ample time for Ms. Pudwill to read her emails, No callback or reply email was received. I purposely waited under the assumption she exercised a common business practice of reading emails first thing in the morning to ensure she was current with activities and correspondence. Maybe, my note was a low priority.

When no answer was forth coming, I called the *Houston Chronicle* "City Desk" and got Ms. Pudwill. I introduced myself and immediately asked whether my email had been read. "No, I sent it on ..." which caused me to ask how she knew where to send it if it hadn't been read. After a long pause, she replied it was my voicemail not the email. I could tell Ms. Pudwill was growing impatient and surly. I asked how interested was she regarding male breast cancer awareness. No answer followed which prompted me to ask how interested was she about women's breast cancer awareness. There was more silence and I sensed she was more inclined to hang up than have a conversation.

Realizing I was getting nowhere with this lady, I requested names of others I could speak with including their phone numbers and whether I could be supplied their email addresses. I was given one phone number and two names:

Todd Ackerman and Mike Hixonbaugh. I emailed them right away and waited until the next day to send a second email via the Houston Chronicle website. I also checked LinkedIn for all three names; Ms. Pudwill and Hixonbaugh were LinkedIn members. I left LinkedIn emails for both of them.

Four days and no replies, later; ample time had passed to read my emails. I called and spoke to Todd Ackerman. He seemed in a hurry to meet several deadlines and gave me little time to discuss MBC. He had me confused with someone else who had supplied him with MBC information the week before in person.

Ackerman believed since the number of MBC incidences were small, there'd be little interest in featuring this disease next month reputed to be women's breast cancer awareness month. I expressed my appreciation for his time and was disappointed with his rejection simply because of the low number of MBC occurrences. I stated there should be some blue in that pink ribbon; to which Mr. Ackerman gave no response. I was assured he'd reply via my email, "soon", but he wasn't specific. Ackerman insisted he was under several deadlines and could not speak, anymore. He never emailed me back.

Well, it got to be mid-October and I had not received word from the *Houston Chronicle* ... again.

Meanwhile, the governor of Texas formally proclaimed the third week in October, 2016, as MBC Awareness Week. Whether this proclamation will apply every year remains to be seen. I saw no such edict in 2017 or 2018.

I've asked over and over, again ... What will it take for the *Houston Chronicle* to publicize MBC awareness?

Female breast cancer awareness is provided ample media coverage throughout the month of October each year while no air time is devoted to male breast cancer. Why? MBC numbers are low; Ackerman concluded there'd be little interest. I fail to understand this decision is strictly based on the number of annual MBC occurrences. What happened to fair and balanced reporting?

Awareness could potentially minimize the risks associated with the disease when early detection signs are known resulting in saved lives. This disease exists, yet, no media believes in launching an awareness campaign. Further, the decision to not publicize MBC awareness appears sexist. Men get this disease, yet, no one wishes to feature or launch a male breast cancer awareness campaign? Breast cancer kills men. What's the solution?

While in search for such an answer, there are proactive measures you and your family can take to ensure this disease will affect fewer men. When a male member of your family reaches manhood, he needs to know what risks his lifestyle choices will determine as he ages. The implications and consequences are self-evident and can be fatal. Do what you can when risks are inconsequential; another practice is to begin disease screenings at an earlier age than 50.

Facebook (FB)

I got this idea since I was on Facebook that I could join an active male breast cancer awareness group. I found one called "The Male Breast Cancer Coalition"; its website seemed credible except for one flawed claim … men have breasts.

I began questioning whether men did have breasts. Herein is what I found and confirmed by breastcancer.org and the MDAnderson Male Breast Cancer Clinic. Before a child of either sex is born, both the male and female are endowed with breast tissue and nipples. When their sex is determined to be female, breasts are formed as the girl matures and enters puberty. Not so with a boy, high testosterone and low levels of estrogen prevents the conversion from breast tissue to breast development. There are two exceptions: when a man has been on steroids or he has become obese. What's more, there have been rare instances where milk ducts have been found in men. Fortunately, due to the male chemical makeup, these milk ducts remained underdeveloped.

After I checked out this website to determine whether I wanted to join, I spoke to a Peggy, a representative of the coalition. The claim that men had breasts bothered me when I knew the contrary; right away, I saw a credibility issue. Nevertheless, our conversation went well in spite of my opposing views about breasts in men and Peggy insisted she wanted to hear my story. I said, "Another time". At the conclusion of this conversation, I was "friended" which granted me access to the "The Male Breast Cancer Coalition" FB postings. However, my "friendship" was short-lived. About a week or so, later, I decided to post my findings about men and breasts on this coalition's page inviting conversation with anyone who had differing views. I was, immediately, "unfriended". Most assuredly, my experience is another example of FB censorship which seemed more important than candid and honest discussion.

What's my conclusion regarding "The Male Breast Cancer Coalition" website Facebook group? Retaining their message that "men have breasts, too" appears to negate fact and truth. For touting a false narrative, they get low grades for integrity and credibility.

Male Cancer Screenings by Age

Refer to the following information obtained from mdanderson.org frequently to ensure you minimize the risks associated with disease. Take a copy with you for your next scheduled examination. This checklist is a guide and dependent on your family history, your doctor. You may therefore wish to alter it, accordingly.

Cancer including MBC is a nasty killer when you allow it to overtake your body before you seek medical attention. Break the male habit of putting off the inevitable; get yourself to your PCP when you're at a lower risk and the disease is still in an early non-invasive stage.

Before Screenings by Age
All Ages

- Speak with you doctor about lung and skin cancer screenings
  - Exams are available for those at increased risk.
- Practice awareness no matter your age below 40
  - Become familiar with your body enough to recognize physiological changes
    - Internal via pain/ inappropriate growths; external
    - Have someone assist you in parts you cannot easily exam (i.e., back,)
    - Report any changes to your doctor without delay

Ages 40-49

- 40: Speak with your doctor about the benefits/limitations of prostate screening and when you should begin testing.
  - 45: Get a digital rectal exam and PSA test every year to check for prostate cancer if you're African American or have a family history (father, brother, son) of prostate cancer.

Ages 50-75

- 50: Have your testosterone and estradiol checked at least once a year to ensue hormonal balance at least once a year
- Get a digital rectal exam and PSA test every year to check for prostate cancer
- Colonoscopy every 10 years or virtual colonoscopy every 5 years to check for colorectal cancer
- 50: Check estrogen level not to exceed 40pg/dL
- 70: Have your estrogen level checked to ensure it's in the healthy range of 21-30pg/dL.

Age 76 and older

- 76: Have your estrogen level checked to ensure it's in the healthy range of 21-30pg/dL.
- 76-85: Discuss with your PCP whether you should continue screening.
  - MD Anderson does not recommend cancer screening for men age 85 and older.

Okay, in spite of all your warnings, precautions, and due diligence, you've discovered an unexplained growth inside your chest usually behind the areola (the dark brown circle that contains your nipple). You're uncertain what it might be; you do know it hurts to the touch and it wasn't there before. Schedule an appointment with your doctor without delay! Do it, Macho-man, before it gets worse!

Don't wait like I did. The mass I found was diagnosed in January, 2011 as a benign gynecomastia. New to this experience, I failed to include a biopsy to validate the diagnosis. Out of ignorance, I blew it off after I heard "benign gynecomastia". I raced to the conclusion it would go away like it did when I was a teenager. I was going to be okay.

Instead, this growth was given all the time it needed to convert and convert it did. Eighteen months later, it was biopsied and diagnosed to be cancerous, stage 3A. I'll always wonder how different the outcome would've been had I taken the time to have the mass removed in 2010 as instructed by my PCP. But, "No!", when I heard "benign", everything was going to be all right! I was spared ... so I thought until that fateful day in late July, 2012."

After you've discovered this growth and scheduled an appointment, the procedure begins with your PCP examination. Based on the findings you may be referred to a breast diagnostic facility for a mammogram, sonogram, ultra-sound, and biopsy. This mass may be simply diagnosed as a benign gynecomastia; good for you, but get it removed right away. Or you'll give this mass ample time to convert to cancer! Remember, all this could have been avoided had you taken the time to get the damn thing removed.

When you make this mistake, staging becomes a significant step. Too, at this point, everything is estimated based the size of the mass, physical condition of your chest, and whether cells were found in your underarm lymph node area.

The next step is surgery followed by a pathology report which more accurately defines the stage of the cancer, tumor size, weight of all tissue removed (chest skin, tumor, breast tissue, underarm lymph nodes, etc.,) whether it's located in one or more areas of your chest or has spread to other parts of the body. The underarm lymph nodes are usually where breast cancer tends to travel, first. Additional blood or imaging tests may be scheduled if there's reason to believe the cancer has spread beyond the breast. Typically, an infusion port is surgically implanted in your chest during the initial surgery to be utilized during post treatment chemo-infusions.

After about a month following surgery, you'll begin weeks of post-cancer treatment. First, there's chemo-therapy; depending on pathology findings you may require one or more phases of chemical infusions. Then, there's radiation treatment intended to stave off recurrence. Lastly, you'll be given an estrogen blocking drug to be taken every day for five years or more, 20mg, orally.

The steps from diagnosis to post treatment explained above are by far simplistic and suggests this experience is nowhere as bad as you might have heard.

Not so fast … Later, I'll describe as accurately as I can how "not so pleasant' this experience became for me. What's more, I've no idea how much damage has been done to healthy tissue and organs in my body from treatment. Chemo infusion, for instance, is indiscriminate; it cannot distinguish healthy vs. unhealthy cells, muscle, fat, or internal organs. At the very least, my body has in many ways prematurely aged due to chemo/radiation therapies. This is another outcome you can avoid should you get an early diagnosis or choose alternative treatment.

If the cancer has spread beyond your chest, you've put off seeking medical attention too long. It's so hard, as it was in my case, to come to terms with what most men deem as a "woman's" disease! Is putting off seeing your PCP a reason or excuse? See your doctor soon after you've discovered an unusual growth in your chest. If you decide the contrary … the consequences are staged below.

Cancer Stages

According to breastcancer.org, cancer staging is defined, numerically, from zero through four. Stage 0 represents a non-invasive cancer that's remained within its original site while stage IV is highly invasive. In this highest stage, the disease has spread from the breast to other parts of the body. Cancer staging characteristics are determined:

- By the size of the mass in centimeters
- Whether the cancer is considered to be invasive or non-invasive
- If the cancer has spread to the underarm lymph nodes
- By how much the cancer has spread to other parts of the body beyond the lymph node and breast areas (metastasized).

Get acquainted with the following medical terms overheard from medical professionals describing the stage of your breast cancer:

- Local: The cancer is confined within the breast.
- Regional: The underarm lymph nodes are involved.
- Distant: The cancer has spread to other parts of the body
- Locally/ Regionally Advanced: The tumor is large and involves the chest skin, underlying chest structures, changes to the breast/ chest/ pectoral shape, and visible lymph node enlargement that can felt during the examination.

Breast cancer staging can help you understand your prognosis (the likely outcome of the disease) and assist your doctor with decisions effecting treatment based on the pathology report findings. Staging gives everyone a common method to describe the breast cancer whose treatment results can be compared and understood relative to other cases.

Stage 0 – A non-invasive breast cancer such as DCIS (ductal carcinoma in situ). There's no evidence that cancer cells or non-cancerous abnormal cells have spread from the originating part of the breast or getting through to or invading adjacent healthy tissue.

Stage I – Invasive breast cancer (Cancer cells breaking through to or invading healthy surrounding breast tissue); Stage I is divided into two subcategories:
- **Stage 1A:**
  - ○ Tumor size $<= 2$ centimeters (cm) AND
  - ○ The cancer has not spread outside the breast-chest area meaning no lymph nodes are involved
- **Stage IB:**
  - ○ No tumor in the breast
    - ▪ Instead, small groups of cancer cells > 0.2 millimeter (mm) and $<= 2$ mm found in the lymph nodes OR

- A tumor is present in the breast <= 2 cm and there are small groups of cancer cells > 0.2 mm and <= 2 mm in the lymph nodes

Microscopic invasion is possible in stage I where the cancer cells have just started to invade the tissue outside the lining of the duct or lobule, but the invading cancer cells are <=1 millimeter.

Stage II – Divided into two subcategories:
- **Stage IIA:**
  - No tumor is found in the breast, but cancer (> 2 mm) is found in 1-3 axillary underarm lymph nodes) or in the lymph nodes near the breast bone (found during a sentinel node biopsy) OR
  - A tumor <= 2 cm has spread to the axillary lymph nodes OR
  - A tumor > 2 cm <= 5 cm has not spread to the axillary lymph nodes

- **Stage IIB:**
  - A tumor > 2 cm and <= 5 cm; small groups of breast cancer cells > 0.2 mm <= 2 mm are found in the lymph nodes OR
  - The tumor > 2 cm <=5 cm; cancer has spread to 1 to 3 axillary lymph nodes or to lymph nodes near the breastbone (found during a sentinel node biopsy) OR
  - A tumor >5 cm that has not spread to the axillary lymph nodes

Stage III – Divided into three subcategories:
- **Stage IIIA:**
  - No tumor is found in the breast or the tumor may be any size; cancer is found in 4-9 axillary lymph nodes or in the lymph nodes near the breastbone (found during imaging tests or a physical exam) OR
  - The tumor > 5 cm; small groups of breast cancer cells (> 0.2 mm <= 2 mm) are found in the lymph nodes OR
  - The tumor > 5 cm; cancer has spread to 1-3 axillary lymph nodes or to the lymph nodes near the breastbone (found during a sentinel lymph node biopsy)
  - A sterling example was my case. As ugly as the left side of my chest looked, the taught/irregular skin, sensitive areola, the ulceration and drainage underneath the puckered nipple, I was still very lucky. I "only" made it to Stage 3A; it had not attached to the chest wall or metastasized. I finally made the time to see the referral surgeon to obtain a prognosis. Putting it

off simply worsened my condition. After surgery, Pathology determined my tumor to be 1.9cm.

- **Stage IIIB:**
  - The tumor may be any size and has spread to the chest wall and/or skin of the breast causing swelling or an ulcer AND
  - May have spread to <= 9 axillary lymph nodes OR
  - May have spread to lymph nodes near the breastbone

- **Stage IIIC:**
  - There may be no sign of cancer in the breast or, if there is a tumor, it may be any size and spread to the chest wall and/or the skin of the breast AND
  - The cancer has spread to 10 or more axillary lymph nodes OR
  - The cancer has spread to lymph nodes above or below the collarbone OR
  - The cancer has spread to axillary lymph nodes or to lymph nodes near the breastbone

Stage IV- Invasive breast cancer that has spread beyond the breast and nearby lymph nodes to other organs of the body: i.e., lungs, distant lymph nodes, skin, bones, liver, or brain.

You may hear the words "advanced" and "metastatic" used to describe stage IV breast cancer. Cancer may be stage IV at first diagnosis or it can be a recurrence of a previous breast cancer that has spread to other parts of the body.

To learn more about treatments generally expected for each stage, cut & paste the following link: breastcancer.org/treatmentplanning/cancerstage

TNM (Tumor, Node, Metastasis) – Is another cancer classification system that may be utilized by your doctor to define your cancer. This system provided more details about the how the cancer looks and behaves. It's based on the tumor size (T), lymph node involvement (N), and whether the cancer has spread (metastasized) to other parts of the body (M).

T (size) category describes the original (primary) tumor:

- **TX** - The tumor can't be measured or found.
- **T0** - There isn't any evidence of the primary tumor.

- **Tis** - The cancer is "in situ" (the tumor has not started growing into healthy breast tissue).
- **T1, T2, T3, and T4:** These numbers are based on the size of the tumor and the extent to which it has grown into neighboring breast tissue. The higher the T number, the larger the tumor and/or the more it may have grown into the breast tissue.

N (lymph node involvement) category describes whether the cancer has reached nearby lymph nodes:

- **NX** means the nearby lymph nodes can't be measured or found.
- **N0** means nearby lymph nodes do not contain cancer.
- **N1, N2, and N3:** These numbers are based on the number of lymph nodes involved and how much cancer is found in them. The higher the N number, the greater the extent of the lymph node involvement.

M (metastasis) category tells whether or not there is evidence that the cancer has traveled to other parts of the body:

- **MX** means metastasis can't be measured or found.
- **M0** means there is no distant metastasis.
- **M1** means that distant metastasis is present.

Once the pathologist knows your T, N, and M characteristics, he/ she can use them to assign a stage to the cancer. For example, a T1 N0 M0 breast cancer would mean that the primary breast tumor is < 2 cm across (T1), has not involved the lymph nodes (N0), and has not spread to distant parts of the body (M0). This cancer would be grouped as stage I.

Provided you can think reasonably well after you've been diagnosed, read Dr. Joseph Mercola's *"The Most Important Steps You Need to Take if You Have Cancer"*. This book is a relevant guide to help those with MBC.

Refer to his website for various articles;
https://articles.mercola.com/sites/articles/archive/2011/02/14/beating-breast-cancer-a-guide-to-prevention-treatment-and-recovery.aspx
The doctor, also, offers natural cancer treatment alternatives.

Support Groups
If you need support, there are such groups available even for men. I've never joined one; however, you can reach out to your cancer treatment facility's Advocacy Groups. There are those strictly for women or men. Support groups

can also be of help for caregivers and those whose family member is fighting this disease and you need to learn more about providing effective support. Attending these types of groups should help you, being a man, to better discuss your concerns with other men and there is comfort knowing you will not be criticized for contracting this disease.

Genetic Testing

It's a good practice to have genetic testing completed shortly after diagnosis or surgery although it can be done at any time. The sooner you know what your genes have afforded you, the better it is to develop a proactive plan to minimize MBC recurrence.

Men with a family history of cancer should request genetic testing to determine whether they, too, carry a gene that might indicate a future recurrence of cancer. It's during this test phase when BRAC mutation testing can be accomplished.

MDAnderson.org and Dr. Mark Lewis, an oncologist at one time for MDA, suggests that before you consider this type of testing, review your family history to obtain relevant information that will be helpful going into the test. You might have a parent or sibling who had cancer before the age of 50. There may be a family history of male/female breast cancer or whether anyone has had two or more cancers at the same time. This type of history might suggest you have a genetic link.

Talk to your counselor and PCP about everything you know concerning your family's medical history; be as specific as possible. A grandparent having died of cancer is good information and can be better when the type of cancer and their age at death is known. Once this history is reviewed, risk factors tailored for you can be discussed.

Determine the usefulness of genetic testing. It cannot accurately predict whether you'll be suitably diagnosed in the future, but will determine whether you're at a greater risk or carrying a gene linked to certain types of cancer. Discuss alternatives with your family. Ask yourself if you'd prefer to deal with a cancer diagnosis or take proactive steps to minimize your cancer exposure, do both or nothing at all? Life is full of choices; it's better to know your future risks following genetic and BRCA testing to plan, accordingly.

Cancer.gov says BRCA1 and BRCA2 mutations are a MBC risk factor. Link http://www.cancer.gov/about-cancer/causes-prevention/genetics/brca-fact-sheet will further your understanding of these genetic mutations. In particular, when BRCA2 mutations are identified, men have close to a 10% lifetime risk they will develop breast cancer.

A big plus and one major difference that men with breast cancer have over women is they respond better to hormone treatment. Approximately 77% of male breast cancers have hormone receptors specific to cancer cell sites where hormones like estrogen can effectively function. Also, 71% of MBCs are BRAC positive (usually BRAC2) which means that male hormonal treatment is likely to be more successful.

Chapter
III
What's It All
About?

General

Yeah, you're probably wondering, "How the hell could I or any man get breast cancer?". Right? I thought that way, too!

Surprise! We can get it depending on a number of circumstances.

Statistics have consistently shown of the approximate 200,000 breast cancer cases in the United States every year, about 0.06 to 1% of breast cancers diagnosed occur in men. In real numbers and this year (2019), the United States can expect 1200 to 2000 MBC cases. Of those diagnosed, here's the deadly part, about 450 men could die from it this and every year. Not good news, is it?

Guess why that number is so high. Typically, men put off seeing a doctor until this cancer is too advanced. You can't fix it, Mr. Handyman! Rearrange your thinking; see your doctor right away!

The likelihood of a man developing breast cancer increases with age. Most male breast cancers are detected between the ages of 60-70 years and include these breast cancer risk factors:

- Family history of breast cancer in a close female relative.
- Abnormal lumps of the breast tissue in response to drug or hormone treatments
- Unusual mass growth due to some infections and poisons
- The development of a mass underneath breast tissue or nipple called a gynecomastia.

There are early signs:
- . A lump is felt underneath the surface of one side of your chest
- The lump grows
- The nipple on that side of your chest is sensitive to pain when accidentally brushed or pressed against
- This lump typically resides behind the areola (the dark brown area) and your nipple
  - That area can become very sensitive to pain when you brush up against it or lean on it
- When such a lump is ignored, a bloody, ulcerated discharge will occur from around the nipple area

Two reasons MBC's uncommon is likely due to the smaller amount of breast tissue in men and there're fewer hormones like estrogen produced in men compared to women (mdanderson.org).

Estrogen

Estrogen, you heard it right! Men have estrogen in our bodies that can be effectively managed before and after it's determined we're in danger of contracting breast cancer. For instance, in Heart Health Guide, http://www.heart-health-guide.com/Aromatase-inhibitors.html, estrogen blockers, aromatase inhibitors (AIs) and estrogen detoxifiers offer a means to fight excess estrogen levels in men. Check into these blockers because they all have side effects and when I take something I want to minimize side effects.

Believe it or don't, estrogen's an important hormone for the man's well-being (mdsnderson.org). When there's an imbalance between testosterone and estrogen over an extended period of time, we run the risk of serious health problems.

Further, there are three types of bioactive estrogens:
- Estrone (E1)
- Estradiol (E2)
- Estriol (E3).

Relative to estradiol, estrone and estriol are far weaker estrogenic estrogen activities with estriol being the weakest. Estrogen's relationship with "T" is further complicated by E2, estradiol. Balance between these estrogen hormones and testosterone defines sexuality in both men and women.

Estradiol is the strongest natural occurring estrogen in men. It can greatly influence male chemistry due to the involvement with the testosterone feedback loop. Estrogens are produced from androgens like testosterone by an enzyme aromatase process that increases with age which promotes the conversion of an androgen (like testosterone) into estradiol. Thus, the older you are, the greater the risk some of your testosterone will be converted (aromatized) into estradiol unless this hormone is periodically monitored to ensure estradiol is in the safety range of 21-30pg/dL for men 60 and older.

Hence, the main biologically active estrogen type in men is *estradiol* (E2). The primary source of estradiol is from the aromatization (Partial conversion to estradiol from "T") of testosterone. As men age, the production of androgens from the adrenals and gonads is on the decline. Testosterone aromatization to estradiol is often maintained, but due to a variety of factors, more "T" is aromatized into fatty tissues, causing a further imbalance between "T" and estrogen, too much estradiol and too little testosterone.

Although, men have very low levels of estrogen in the pica range (that's 1×10 to the -12th power), any high estrogen levels (>30pg/dL.) can create complications in men as it does in women (cancer.gov). However, there are estrogen blockers, aromatase inhibitors, and estrogen detoxifiers considered to be natural solutions to prevent the completion of the aromatase process. As might be surmised, a high estrogen level increases the risk of prostate problems, low libido, male breast cancer, short stature, and gynecomastia in men.

Dr. Shippen, an anti-aging researcher and author of *The Testosterone Syndrome*, believes that "men's bodies would not have a process for making estrogen if it were useless to them." He identifies many estrogen-sensitive areas of the male body such as the brain and explains that estrogen is an extremely important aspect of the brain chemistry that triggers natural sexual functions. He goes on to say, "Too little estrogen will neuter a man just as effectively as too little testosterone."

On the other hand, for most adult men, the problem is not too little estrogen, it's having too much! A primary cause of hormone imbalance in men as they age is that "T" is increasingly converted to estrogen resulting in an excess of estradiol. *Life Extension* magazine recommends men maintain estradiol levels between 21.8 and 30.1 pg/dL.

Similar to how women react to small amounts of testosterone, men have a very small window of optimal effectiveness regarding estrogen. Since estrogen is derived from aromatase, it actually displaces testosterone at the receptor sites which essentially "turns off" testosterone-driven activities. Thus, estrogen and "T" exist in a delicate balance. What's more, this imbalance, I believe, can precipitate the development of a benign gynocomastia when left unattended to grow will eventually convert into a cancerous tumor … like mine did.

While men need estrogen to make sexuality possible, it can, also, act as an on/off switch stuck in the off position. As Dr. Shippen puts it, "Like so many things that work well when we are young, the control mechanism aspect of estrogen can get out of hand as we grow older. Illness, drugs, dietary imbalances, lifestyle, and certain aspects of normal aging help accelerate this process and raise estrogen levels to unhealthy heights."

Common causes of elevated estrogen in men are:
- Age-related increase in aromatase activity
- Changes in liver function

- Obesity
- Alcohol abuse
- Drug abuse (amphetamines, marijuana, or cocaine)
- Zinc deficiency
- Ingestion of estrogen-enhanced foods or substances
- Drug-related estrogen imbalances (e.g., over-the-counter pain relievers and anti-inflammatories re: ibuprofen, acetaminophen, and aspirin; antibiotics; anti-fungal drugs; cholesterol-lowering drugs; anti-depressants and anti-psychotics; heart and blood pressure medicines; antacids; and some vitamins, nutrients, and foods rich in vitamin E and grapefruit).

These problems are typically interrelated; men frequently have more than one estrogen-heightening influence. To complicate matters, the male body's built-in methods to eliminate estrogen can waver which adds to the excess.

An article in *Life Extension* magazine November 2008 By William Faloon stresses the dangers of excessive estrogen in an aging male and how these high levels can occur as men age.

An interesting side-effect of elevated male estrogen is it can trick the brain into believing your "T" supply is adequate which will slow the natural production of testosterone. What's more, the combination of low "T" and high estrogen can be particularly dangerous. There's an increased risk of male heart attack or stroke and this condition adversely affects the prostate gland. Fortunately, this hormonal imbalance can be successfully treated with hormone therapy.

As men age, the amount of "T" produced in the testes significantly decreases while estradiol levels increase. The reason for this condition is an increase in the aromatase activity combined with age-associated fat mass, especia4lly about the belly. It appears the estradiol levels correlate with subcutaneous body fat. The greater this type of fat and fat accumulates about the abdomen, the more likely most of your "T" was converted to estradiol. Further, aging men with abdominal obesity seem to be more susceptible to degenerative disorders like heart disease, diabetes, and cancer.

A man's waist circumference is an accurate measurement of future disease risk. Excess estradiol secretion is at least one of the deadly processes associated with the challenges of having too much abdominal fat.

Symptoms of excess estrogen in aging men include:

- Development of breasts
- Excessive abdominal fat
- Feeling run-down
- Muscle mass loss
- Becoming overly emotional

Many of these symptoms can, also, be linked to a testosterone deficiency.

Testosterone

Every guy has it, "T", that is. Most everyone defines testosterone as the essence of maleness and manliness. It makes men feel, look, and perform better, physically and sexually. Nevertheless, most people would be surprised that estrogen also plays a key role in men's sexuality. Moreover, it's essential to their cardiovascular and circulatory health, their muscle mass and bone strength.

Whereas women need a small amount of testosterone, men need a small bit of estrogen. These minute quantities of opposing hormones complement each other while they portray a delicate hormonal balance affecting the man's physical, emotional well-being, and sexual health.

So, what does "T" do for men? First, the effect of testosterone in men's health can be grouped into two categories: *androgenic* and *anabolic*. Androgenic refers to the growth of facial and body hair, sex organ development, deepening of the voice, and male pattern baldness. The anabolic effects stimulate the growth of muscle, bone, and red blood cells.

Testosterone affects the man's brain, voice, hair, muscles and fat, organs, bones, and libido. What's more, the effects of "T" on these body systems differ during each stage of his life.

When in the fetal stage, testosterone and dihydrotestosterone (DHT) are necessary in the formation of internal and external male genitalia. During puberty, "T" deepens the voice, prompts the growth of facial and body hair, stimulates sexual behavior, and begins the production of sperm.

Adult male "T" is necessary to maintain muscle mass and strength, bone density, normal hair growth, libido, and sperm production.

With all that's going on in the adult male body, how does anyone determine what's "normal"? A healthy adult male's "T" range is between 348-

1197ng/dL (nanograms per deciliter) of blood plasma. Due to this broad range, it can become a challenge to detect an excess or deficiency.

Life Extension believes that a "moderately youthful" range between 700-900 ng/dL should be considered adequate or optimal for manliness. However, each person's body chemistry is different. What might seem low for one may be adequate for another and vice-versa. It depends on lifestyle, activity, diet, stress, age, and so many other attributes. Thus, "normal" is relative to the individual male and his lifestyle choices. Further, testosterone is released about eight times each day for most adult males. A peak release occurs around 8 AM while the lowest occurs about 10 pm in the evening. Furthermore, male "T" release appears to not coincide with a lunar or monthly cycle as some people might surmise.

To determine normalcy for an adult male is critical in (testosterone replacement therapy) TRT. What's important and usually non-existent is a normal, healthy chemical baseline of the male patient. Most often it's unavailable for his doctor to refer before an irregularity is detected. Moreover, the average age-related decline in male testosterone is slow which adds to the complexity to determine patient normalcy. Plus, a hormonal imbalance is dependent on the patient's age, activity, severity of the decline or excess, physical condition, and length of time this imbalance has existed. That's why it's essential to have periodic visits with your PCP when you are well to establish "norms" in your blood work and vitals for future use.

There are bound to be hormonal changes as men age and they typically begin at just before they reach the 40 year mark. However, just as women can begin menopause at an earlier age, so can men experience andropause (male menopause) sooner as well.

Here's a serious consideration regarding men and breast cancer. Between the ages of 25 and 50, testosterone decreases by about 50%. It gets closer to the 50% mark when you choose a sedentary lifestyle. At the same time, estrogen levels, specifically estradiol, increase by approximately the same percentage which potentially exposes men to hormonal imbalance and disease especially male breast cancer.

A "T" deficiency can be associated with a number of possible symptoms which can lead to misdiagnosis or these symptoms cannot be explained at all. Some medical professionals believe when there's a chronic or recurring condition, a hormonal deficiency should be considered when searching for the cause. Hormonal imbalance is good to remember when seeking advice from your PCP; you could mention this possible reason for the way you're feeling.

Testosterone affects the body in many ways. Deficiency symptoms include changes in physical characteristics, the cardiovascular & circulatory system, mental & emotional states of mind, and sexual dysfunction. A number of the following factors can, also, accelerate "T" deficiencies in the aging man:

- Excess weight
- Extraordinary amount of abdominal fat
- Insulin resistance
- Low HDL cholesterol
- Low bone density
- Illness or disease
- Stressful events
- Depression or mental illness
- Reduced sexual activity.

These very factors can be the cause as well as an effect of a "T" deficiency and estradiol excess. Thus, establishing "normalcy" in men can be challenging; everyone's chemical makeup is different.

Physical Characteristics
Adult males go through physical changes as they grow older; many of them can be attributed to the age-related "T" decline. They might include loss of body hair and baldness, a decrease in muscle mass while accumulating more body fat which will affect strength and physical capabilities. They can also experience a reduction in energy and stamina. To add to the decline is your metabolic rate, that's the rate at which you burn calories. It slows down especially when you choose not to include an exercise program in your lifestyle. Although, these changes may be considered part of "normal" aging, they can be accelerated by a "T" deficiency (except your metabolism; it can slow down even more the less active you become.). This decline in "T" can be somewhat slowed when undergoing testosterone replacement therapy.

What is likely to happen with low "T", an inactive lifestyle, and a slow metabolic rate? You can put on body fat that much easier.

Cardiovascular
Since testosterone is a muscle-building hormone and the heart is a muscle, low "T" levels can lead to cardiovascular disease. According to the November 1999 issue of *Life Extension Magazine*, "Testosterone is not only responsible

for maintaining heart muscle protein synthesis, but it is a promoter of coronary dilation and helps to maintain healthy cholesterol levels". A deficiency can lead to:

- Elevated blood pressure
- Increased insulin levels
- Increased cholesterol and triglycerides
- Diminished coronary artery elasticity
- Weakening of the heart muscle
- Increased abdominal fat, which further increases the risk of a heart attack.

Mental

Mental and emotional problems associated with a "T" deficiency can often be overlooked (especially when most men are reluctant to discuss those issues). Nonetheless, they can be devastating. *Life Extension* reports the following potential mental issues resulting from low "T" levels:

- Mood swings/overly emotional
- Easy irritability
- Tendency to be timid
- Inner unrest
- Loss of interest in most anything
- Inability to concentrate
- Memory loss
- Reduced intellectual agility
- Passive attitudes
- Overall tiredness
- Feelings of weakness
- Hypochondria.

Note these symptoms, can also be associated with depression and usually can be relieved with testosterone therapy.

Sexual

Testosterone is the key to male sexuality. In his book, *The Testosterone Syndrome*, Dr. Eugene Shippen explains that, "In fact, all the different structural components of the genital area-nerves, arteries, veins, muscles - are guided in their formation by testosterone and maintained in good, working order, throughout life, by that very same hormone."

Except, sexuality is far more complex; it gets complicated due to several interrelated factors. Testosterone affects the brain, influencing sexual interest, attraction, and arousal besides sexuality. In *Super "T"*, Dr. Karlis Ullis explains what hormonal effects can have on:

1. **Sexual interest** (libido) - Related to spikes in "T" levels reaching brain receptors.
2. **Attraction and arousal** - Linked to male/female body odors called pheromones. A male with low testosterone will no longer be as pungent after a workout.
3. **Sexual receptivity** - Is related to sexual function for men and not cyclical.
4. **Sexual function** - For men is surprisingly less dependent on "T" as it is on nitric oxide, which keeps the blood vessels in the penis open for erections.
5. **Sexual pleasure** *and sensitivity* - Are heightened when testosterone levels peak.
6. **Sexual orgasm** - Is enhanced by testosterone.
7. **Sexual fulfillment** - Is accomplished by the rise in oxytocin (A hormone in the hypothalamus part of the brain, transported to and secreted by, the pituitary gland). Oxytocin is enhanced by estrogen and antagonized by a high "T" level.
8. **Sexual bonding** (or love and marriage) - Mediated in men by testosterone. It works by activating the pituitary hormone vasopressin which causes men to pursue women and become territorial.

Picture how easy a sex hormonal imbalance can affect male sexuality. One of the first signs of a "T" deficiency is in your libido. A lowered desire can lead to difficulties with sexual function and fulfillment. Further complications can follow because low testosterone is often related to a man's sense of overall well-being and self-worth. Thus, sexual problems can contribute to mental or emotional problems (i.e., low self-esteem, moodiness, and depression), which can compound sexual problems. What's more, without treatment this cycle would continue.

Gynecomastia
Men should become aware of a common male breast condition known as gynecomastia. It's not a form of cancer, nevertheless, it does cause a growth under the nipple or areola (the brownish area that surrounds the nipple) that can be felt and seen depending on how much it protrudes. Further, the area where it resides can be painful to the touch when leaned against or brushed by it.

At the same time, the size of this lump under the nipple could be a potential onset of male breast cancer. All it takes is time to allow it to grow larger. Smart men will get it diagnosed right away while it remains a benign gynecomastia. Then, have it surgically removed right away.

Other symptoms of MBC include nipple inversion, pain, bleeding or skin ulceration. If you're "nursing" such a growth, see a doctor at once!

In my case, this lump grew ever so slowly, caused some protrusion, and began to interfere with my workouts. If I pressed that part of my chest against an exercise bench or even accidentally brushed it, I felt a sharp pain from my areola to the base of my tongue lasting for several seconds. It was a pain so excruciating I'd never experienced anything like it before!

Teenage boys can get a gynecomastia quite often due to hormonal changes during adolescence. It happened to me and after my examination; our GP concluded it would eventually go away. This experience was supposed to be part of puberty and it did just what our doctor said; it went away.

Except, what I didn't know was older men can get this growth due to late-life hormonal swings which ultimately results in hormonal imbalance. What's more, certain medications and some conditions like Klinefelter syndrome can cause a gynecomastia to develop.
Although, it's rare, a gynecomastia can form as an unusual mass below your skin line inside your chest. It's most common behind your nipple. No matter where it forms in your chest get to your doctor without delay. There's always the risk it's a precursor to cancer. The sooner you have this growth biopsied, the better your chances are you know what it is and what can be done about it before it gets complicated. Get this mass removed!

And men, here's where I made my mistake! I treated this late life growth in my chest like I did as a teenager. It was a mass that would eventually go away. Instead, due to my ignorance, it got larger and converted to cancer.

According to the *Journal of National Cancer Institute*, February 19, 2014, if a man develops a gynecomastia late in life, it has a tenfold chance of converting to cancer (When you give it enough time to grow as in my case!). Once you discover such a mass, get it removed as quickly as you can to reduce the risk of getting cancer.

In spite of data and studies, it's believed that having a gynecomastia form is not supposed to be a precancerous condition. However, when hormonal changes (i.e., an increase in estrogens and decrease of androgens) occur, a gynecomastia can form in advanced aged adult men. The danger lies when you put off having this mass diagnosed and allow the lump time to become cancerous. How would you know this information? How would your doctor know of any hormonal imbalance? Awareness and testing is the answer, except most men and doctors don't know or test for hormonal changes in men. It's a mistake and has to change!

My experience clearly illustrated my ignorance and consequence. Virtually ignoring the presence of a mass in my chest increased my risk of developing breast cancer by ten times! If you develop such a tumor or notice an unusual growth, get it examined immediately! No more macho-man putting it off, here!

Tissue or Breast?
When men think of breast cancer, they most often view it strictly as a disease affecting women. To validate this notion, men see significant anatomical differences between the sexes which reinforces their conviction they cannot get breast cancer. For instance, an adult women's breast tissue has milk ducts, lobules and functional epithelial cells whereas men do not. Since women have more breast tissue and they are chemically different, men believe they will be exempt from acquiring this disease.

As odd as it may seem, male breast tissue develops the same way as in women. In fact, adult male breast tissue is similar to a girl's breasts before puberty according to webmd.com. They consist of a few lesser developed ducts than are developed in girls. During puberty, hormonal changes in the girl cause her breast tissue to grow into breasts whereas male hormones produced by the testicles prevent breast growth in teenage boys.

Moreover, MBC can begin in the ducts and spread into surrounding cells just like the ladies. Although rare, men can develop Paget's disease of the nipple. This condition happens when a tumor that began in a duct beneath the nipple moves to the surface. Male breasts have fewer lobules if they have any at all; therefore, lobular carcinoma seldom occurs in men.

Nevertheless, as uncommon as it may seem, breast tissue is still breast tissue and men are as susceptible to the disease as women (http://www.webmd.com/breast-cancer/). Further, men can get the same types of breast cancers women can with few exceptions. Where cancers involve breast milk producing and storing regions, men are anatomically unequipped to acquire this type of breast cancer.

Men argue they do not have breasts unless, of course, they're obese. It sounds too feminine to make that claim and under ordinary circumstances, the closest a man can get to having breasts is they have breast tissue. Whether you're obese or lean, part of your chest is composed of this breast tissue. As embarrassing as it may seem, get over it! Surrender to the reality even though it sounds un-masculine. Admit it out loud; you have breast tissue.

To clear more possible confusion about breast vs. chest, understand, first, I'm a guy, a proud, straight guy who knows only obese men possess what appear to be breasts. Except these supposed breasts are merely made up of fat tissue. Every male has breast tissue in his chest wall and dependent on your body's fat percent, you'll either appear to have a chest or a chest with a set of breasts. Lean or otherwise, you'll always have a chest with breast tissue sans the woman's anatomical version of a breast.

Here is, yet, another misunderstanding. Breast cancer is considered a woman's disease because of the extremely low incident rate in men, one percent or less per year in the United States. Due to the low numbers, little is done to ensure MBC awareness is known. Most male breast cancer begins in cells lining the ducts. It's very rare and usually affects older men in the 60-70 age range. Since men have a low rate of the disease, MBC is typically found in later stages when the disease is more difficult to treat and manage.

According to my MDA cancer team and mdanderson.org, male breast cancer occurs when malignant cells form in the breast tissue. Any man can develop breast cancer; it's just more common among older men when the release of "T" is on the decline while estrogen is on the rise.

Cancercenter.com says in view of a variety of breast cancer types, every case needs to be evaluated to determine the best method of treatment by your PCP. First, the mass has to be located and analyzed. Did the disease spread to other parts of the body (metastasize) from the breast? Dependent on your physician's findings, your cancer will be categorized according to severity, i.e., stage 1C, stage 3A, and so on.

The cause of MBC is said to be not known according to several cancer treatment facilities including MDAnderson. Risk factors include a family history of breast cancer, prior radiation exposure, and having acquired Klinefelter syndrome.

I'd add two more risk factors: lifestyle choices and hormonal imbalance. Even though obesity may increase a man's risk of contracting breast cancer, in many instances, it's unclear, according to most literature, what causes the disease. I disagree and believe it's largely due to hormonal imbalance.

One of the largest studies conducted until February 19, 2014 collected data from independent studies of about 2,400 men with breast cancer and 52,000 men who did not have the disease. These common risk factors associated with MBC were confirmed: obesity, Klinefelter syndrome (a rare genetic condition), and gynecomastia.

Scientists at the National Cancer Institute (NCI) pooled risk factor data from over 21 studies of male breast cancer cases. The results of this collaboration appeared on Feb. 19, 2014, in the *Journal of National Cancer Institute* and posted on the cancer.gov website.

Scientists, led by Louise Brinton, Ph.D., and Michael B. Cook, Ph.D., NCI, concluded men were at greater risk for breast cancer with a high body mass index (BMI). Men with the highest BMI had a 35% greater risk of breast cancer compared to men with a lower BMI. This elevated risk in men with a high BMI (typically had excess breast tissue and higher estrogen levels) appeared similar to postmenopausal women for breast cancer risk.

Get this, in the same study, a gynecomastia presence, independent of Klinefelter syndrome and obesity, was associated with a 10-fold increased risk of breast cancer in men when the mass was not removed right away.

In simpler terms, when a lump is found in your chest usually around the areola, get to your doctor without delay. If the biopsy identifies it as a benign gynecomastia, have it removed inside a month's time to be on the safe side. Deciding the converse like I did and allowing it to grow will increase your risk by ten times that it will convert to cancer. This moment is one of the few times in your life when immediate action is essential!

The blunder I made when I heard "benign" was I thought it would go away like it did when I was a teenager. Big mistake! Instead, I gave it ample time to become cancerous and that oversight haunts me every day of my life! Don't make the same mistake!

Survival
If you've been diagnosed, you want to know whether you'll survive. Survival rates vary for male breast cancer; stage for stage they're the same as in women. However, men typically wait for medical evaluation at a later stage. Men with the BRCA2 gene mutation, Li-Fraumeni syndrome, Klinefelter

syndrome, Cowden syndrome or a family history of breast cancer are at an increased risk for breast cancer.

I'm a first-rate example of putting it off. Out of ignorance, hope what I had this time would act as it did when in my teens, I let the damn thing grow and convert into stage three MBC.

An MDA study found on mdanderson.org, the five year overall survival rate for MBC was just 63%. This low rate hinges on how receptive a MBC survivor is to making lifestyle changes. With better choices, not only will the survival rate go up, he will potentially extend his life.

When a man develops breast cancer, his female relatives are at a higher risk of contracting the disease. In fact, the risk is highest when the man carries a BRAC mutation described earlier.

The lifetime risk for men to get MBC is estimated to be one in 1,000 men. Risk factors include family members of either gender who's had breast cancer, a genetic condition associated with high estrogen levels, chronic liver disorders, alcoholism, and obesity. The older the man becomes, the more susceptible he is to the disease dependent on genes and lifestyle choices.

MBC Treatment Alternatives
Okay, it turns out you were one of the unfortunate few who's acquired breast cancer. Treatment typically consists of the removal of the affected skin including the areola, tumor, and breast tissue followed by one or more phases of chemotherapy, radiation, hormonal therapy, and/or other targeted therapies. How much post-cancer treatment is prescribed depends on what extent you've the disease and stage you, finally, figured out it was time to see your doctor.

If the cancer has been confined to the chest area, adjuvant therapy similar to what women go through will be followed after surgery. On the other hand, when the disease has spread to the lymph nodes and beyond, chemo, radiation, and, possibly, other therapies will become necessary. Since many MBCs are hormone receptor-positive, the use of the drug Tamoxifen is frequently a standard therapy for men; expect to be on this drug for at least five years.

Here's what happens after surgery. All removed material (skin, areola, tumor, breast tissue, and lymph nodes) is weighed and sent to pathology for analysis. You'll be expected to stay until the next day after surgery. Meanwhile, a formal report is issued to the recovering cancer treatment team assigned to you. It can become an anxious time until the results are known and usually takes about a day or your first post-surgery visit several days later. Part of the analysis will include a DNA number; the lower the value, the lower your risk percentage of MBC recurrence for the next 20 years.

Chapter
IV
Back to Balance

General

Conclusions in this chapter are strictly from substantiated research and my personal experience without medical training; I'm, by no means, a doctor. I believe many of the MBC cases could have been prevented IF what I'm proposing is universally implemented. Further, I say there are several areas men need to focus proactively to minimize the risks associated with contracting this disease.

First, it's important that men view themselves, differently. Back off on the sense of invincibility or macho attitude; realize you're human and you can get this disease. Believe it or don't, whether you contract any disease depends on how well you've managed your life with few exceptions I'll explain later.

There are nine contributing factors that determine how effectively disease is managed as we age. Disease management hinges on your awareness and willingness to make necessary changes intended to minimize your exposure to any sort of disease including cancer

As we age, we become comfortable and complacent with our chosen lifestyle. Heck, you're typically over 40 years of age and you've a long life ahead with most of the drudgery behind. Typically, you're less physically active and oft times bend the rules of good health. But you're all grown up, now; you don't need anyone telling you what to do, right, Macho-man? The first major step you can take is getting over yourself!

Now, let's examine these nine characteristics of sensible disease management that just might change your mind:
- Genes
- Age
- Lifestyle
- Diet
- Supplementation
- Adequate, uninterrupted, quality sleep
- Effective coping skill sets to manage anxiety and stress
- Exercise
- Hormonal balance

Two of the above traits, we have no control: genes and age. Whatever you've inherited from family cannot be changed by science as we know it, today. Genes make up of about 30% of life extension opportunity. Surprisingly, they're responsible for a mere 5% of cancers. The real culprits are mostly:

poor diet, living a sedentary lifestyle, and hormonal imbalance, Age? Once the engine starts, science can slow it down, but cannot stop or reverse it, yet.

The remaining seven, we can manage contingent on your willingness to do it sans drugs. It's healthier without prescribed medicines. Side effects from prolonged drug use are eliminated and your liver will not have to work as hard when you aren't on prescribed meds. Nevertheless, it's a lifestyle choice to decide what you're willing to do to regain your health and stay that way.

Before we get into each of these factors, I'd emphasize the importance of annual check-ups to ensure you're effectively doing what you can to prevent disease. In fact, after 49, make these annual check-ups more like semi-annual. Good health can only be determined by periodic examinations. Starting at age 50 and thereafter, be certain you see your PCP at least twice a year. These semi-annual examinations are a must, no exceptions!

Diet
Eating a healthy, balanced diet is important for prolonged energy and illness prevention. Eating healthy is far from just cutting calories or strict dieting. Rather, it's to ensure your body gets the nutrition it needs to thrive and feel alive. The expression," Full of energy and ready to go!" has been embraced for a long time. I feel exactly that way after a good sleep and nutritious breakfast.

Be aware of calories and avoid the intent to cut them, just don't consume as many. Pay more attention to resistant starch calories. Healthy and active adults need about 2,000 calories a day. The more exercise you do, the more calories you use. A daily calorie calculator (Go online to find one.) can be utilized to determine how many calories you need each day. Keep in mind, you only burn up to 30% of your total daily calories when you hit the gym; in most instances, it's closer to 10-15%. Therefore, you've got to learn to move and move often.

Add fruits and vegetables to every meal. They're better to snack on, too. Add a banana or dried cranberries or blueberries to your cereal at breakfast or why not add all three? Eat a salad and an apple at lunchtime. Have some tomatoes and fruit with your dinner. This way, you can get the recommended minimum three to five servings of fruit and vegetables each day.

Try some new foods. When you go to the grocery store, purposely, find something in produce you've never eaten before. It can only help steer you towards a healthier, more balanced diet, plus, you won't get bored eating the same foods all the time.

Check out your portions; the more appropriate they are can make a big difference. One means is to read the nutrition label for recommended serving sizes.

Salt, different sugars, caffeinated and alcoholic drinks in excess are toxic to the body. Notwithstanding, excessive alcohol can do serious damage to your liver. Eat a healthy, well balanced diet by reducing your intake of these edibles. Note, a sugar is any ingredient ending in "…ose" (ex., dextrose, sucrose, etc.).

Clean your home of junk-out, foodless foods. If the temptation isn't there you're less likely to eat it, especially at nighttime. When you're able to cut these foods out (sugary, salty snacks), you'll eat what's available in your home instead. And what you have in the balance should be healthy such as fruits, vegetables, nuts, and whole grains.

Balance your diet with proteins and carbohydrates. Include meats, beans and fish for protein. I eat mostly sea foods and poultry. Avoid cutting out carbohydrates because they're needed for energy. Fruits, vegetables, whole grains, multi-grain breads, and wheat pasta contain those necessary carbohydrates.

And if you're 40 or more, you might consider eating lower glycemic index (GI) foods. The magic number is to eat foods whose GI is 50 or lower (sugar/sugar products have a GI of close to or equal to 100). Research online for more details about GI and GI mean.

Drink more water, preferably tap water instead of a soda or beer. Keep drinking bottled water to a minimum; it's less regulated than tap water. You, also, run the risk of taking in micro-plastics when drinking bottled water. Besides, tap water is free or, at least, less expensive if you have a water bill.

Chew food thoroughly. Rushing a meal is not healthy and you tend to eat more when you gulp it down. A must is to always have a healthy breakfast. Late-night snacks are a no-no; eat with purpose rather than pleasure, alone.

I've never gone on any of those popularized diets to lose weight. I've always had the discipline to make sure my waist size was under control. What I've read in years past is that fad dieting can be unhealthy. It's better to reduce your daily food intake by about 100 calories and through the course of 12 months or so, you could expect to lose about ten pounds. It means, though, you're going to have to take the time to count calories; write them down, and track them. When you increase your output as in exercise or activity, you're likely to lose more weight, sooner. Thus, the combination of calorie reduction and increased activity will result in a leaner you in a shorter length of time.

Independent studies agree that when you fill your dinner plate with two-thirds color (fruits & vegetables) and one third your choice of meat, preferably fowl, buffalo, wildlife meats, or fish, you've a nutritious selection for your meal. MDAnderson, however, encourages you to fill your plate with three-fourths color which has been my choice since 2012.

As we advance in age, be acutely concerned about saturated fats and taking in too many simple carbohydrate foods especially after dinner. Simple carbs will put on fat when you fail to work the calories off. I attempt to eat my simple carbohydrates earlier in the day when I've a greater chance of burning them off.

A reminder regarding diet is how metabolism changes as we age. I talked about this in Chapter III.

Fasting

Have you ever considered fasting between your evening meal and breakfast (No snacking after your evening meal.)? Here's a study that may be of interest. Caution: The study may appear skewed since it excludes men. Candy Sagon wrote the article in the AARP Daily News Alert on April 04, 2016. It says fasting at night may lower breast cancer recurrence in women who've survived early stage breast cancer. Since the MBC rate is so low, men were excluded from the study. Even so, fasting could reduce risks of recurrence for everyone who've survived early stage breast cancer.

In addition to researchers emphasizing what cancer survivors should eat, this study exclaims it may have to do with how much they don't eat after their evening meal. Also, the study stressed the importance of time between the last meal of the day and when breakfast was eaten.

What's more, I say this same practice could very well be beneficial to prevent breast cancer, altogether. Read the entire source article to determine whether a 13 hour fast could be added to your lifestyle as a proactive means of prevention.

The study, itself, was published March 31, 2017 in *JAMA Oncology*, and found that not eating for 13 hours between dinner and breakfast could help reduce the risk of recurrence in women with early-stage breast cancer. Although, it's unclear why fasting would have this effect, researchers noted that with every additional two hours of fasting, the average blood sugar in women decreased while their hours of sleep increased. Since quality sleep went up while glucose was lowered, the risk associated with disease was minimized.

There were 2,413 women in the study comprised of ladies between 27 to 70 years of age who were not diabetic, but diagnosed with early-stage breast cancer. With seven years follow-up, the study concluded that women who fasted less than 13 hours overnight had a 36% greater risk for breast cancer recurrence compared with those who fasted more than 13 hours. Furthermore, there appeared to be no link between a shorter fasting time and death from breast cancer or other diseases.

"Among generally healthy adults, there are no apparent risks of extending the nightly fasting interval and it could potentially improve metabolic health and/or sleep patterns," author Ruth Patterson of the University of California, San Diego told AARP via email. She believes the findings are "too premature" to publicly recommend this healthy practice would prevent cancer recurrence.

Anti-Cancer Specific Spices and Foods
According to Chris Wark's SquareOne Modules, these items are the top cancer fighters/preventers. What I've listed are strictly what I've selected to eat and not an all-inclusive Chris Wark list of recommendations.
- Cayenne, turmeric, curcumin, garlic
- Pumpkin and sunflower seeds
- Mixed, deluxe nuts, preferably unsalted
- Broccoli sprouts
- Watercress
- Celery
- Beets
- Carrots
- Broccoli
- Cauliflower
- Onions

- White button, Shitake, and Portabella Mushrooms. They should be cooked before eaten. I sauté them in olive oil before I put them in my salad.
- Berries of any variety: blackberries, cranberries, raspberries, strawberries
- Bananas
- Apples
- And, for grins, watermelon (I don't know of its anti-cancer qualities.)

With regard to vegetables, the emphasis is on raw, raw veggies. Fix yourself a large bowl of this vegetable salad without salad dressing and eat it twice a day (lunch and dinner) to help heal you from or prevent cancer. You can vary its contents each time you make it; you don't have to have the same ingredients each time the salad is made. The salad will be a bit chewy and its flavor is more pleasant than you might think.

If you need to add more flavor, mix water with lemon juice (About half and half, I never measure.) as a dressing.

I refrain from red meat, but will eat buffalo over beef (About two or three times a month). I focus on seafood (salmon, trout, scallops, shrimp or two-legged meats; chicken, turkey.

I eat fruit several times a day, generally, at least four types of "berries" and typically three bananas throughout the day. They can be eaten during or between meals.

For added flavor when eating bananas or apples, I will occasionally top them with crunchy peanut butter. Ymmmm …

Stay away from all processed foods, breads, desserts, anything sugary like "sugarless" foods or chewing gums, and alcohol. Remember cancer loves sugar!

Supplementation
Before you say anything, you may very well not want to take supplements at all. On the other hand, you cannot possibly take in all nutrients your body needs from the food you eat. What's more, I've placed supplements under diet because I consider them an additional source of nutrition necessary for your health and longevity. Whatever supplements you choose, they're better absorbed right after a meal.

For me, I've found supplementation has effectively worked for over 50 years of my life. Yes, in spite of what I've taken for so long, I still contracted cancer. More on that subject, later. Meanwhile, you decide what you will or will not take to supplement what you eat.

Below, I've listed a number of supplements I take for reasons explained. If you still have doubts, surf the Net; webmd.com is a good source to obtain answers.

Because I lead a very active life via resistance exercise and interval training on the bike/treadmill a week at a moderate to high intensity level five to six days, my system requires more supplementation than the "average bear". Refer to my notations for the supplements I take to maintain my lifestyle.

A word about "minimum daily requirements" … This standard was determined by utilizing a 150lb. sedentary 50 year old man as the model many years ago. Things have changed. Moreover, your age and activity will determine your personal daily supplementation requirement.

Acetyl L-Carnitine - **250 mg**
This amino acid has shown to improve memory in elderly people. It helps treat male infertility caused by inflammation of some reproductive organs and tissues (prostrate, seminal vesicles, and epididymis). The symptoms of age-related testosterone deficiency ("male menopause") can be relieved by utilizing this product. Since it improves blood flow to the brain, memory can be enhanced.

It also converts fats to energy and boosts antioxidant activity in the body. When taken as a supplement, it can protect the brain from stress caused by alcohol and aging. In a 2006 study, people who were given 1,000 milligrams (mg) of acetyl L-carnitine a day experienced relief from mild chronic depression.

Alpha Lipoic Acid (ALA)
There has been sparse research on this antioxidant compound (webmd.com). There is some evidence that ALA may have at least two positive benefits for those with type 2 diabetes. Few studies have suggested that ALA may improve one's ability to use its own insulin to lower blood sugar with type 2 diabetics. It may also help reduce nerve damage that may have been caused by this disease.

Some people use alpha-lipoic acid for memory loss, chronic fatigue syndrome (CFS), HIV/AIDS, cancer, liver disease, diseases of the heart and blood vessels (including a disorder called cardiac autonomic neuropathy) and Lyme disease.

Alpha-lipoic acid is also used to treat eye-related disorders, such as damage to the retina, cataracts, glaucoma, and an eye disease called Wilson's disease.

Note there's a combined acetyl L-carnitine/alpha lipoic acid capsule on the market which I prefer to use when it's available. I take the combined supplement twice a day, once after breakfast and after dinner in the evening.

Vitamin B3-Niacinamide
According to the Pierce-Shaw book, *Life Extension*, you can modify your desire to eat sweets by altering your blood sugar regulation. Changing how you feel about eating foods is better than resorting to will power and deprivation. Niacinamide, a form of B3, has been used to treat hypoglycemia. A sufficient dose allows blood sugar to rise and stabilize, but it's not enough to stimulate the release of insulin or cause it to become abnormally high.

A five year study of 1000 cardiovascular male patients taking three grams of niacin each day to lower serum cholesterol and triglycerides had surprising results. Niacin slowed the removal of sugar from their blood. It, also, reduced their appetites which caused weight loss.

I take it for the very reasons explained, above. I wanted to minimize my urge to eat sweets and it seems to work. I split my dosage of 500 mg at each meal time and double the dosage when my cravings appear to be overwhelming.

Now that I'm in my 80s, I'm finding my sweet cravings have subsided or maybe it's because I've had this discipline for so long, I don't get the level of cravings I used to get. Thus, I haven't had to rely so much on this supplement.

Vitamin B12
In a British study, older people with the lowest levels of B12 lost brain volume at a faster rate over a span of 5 years than those with the highest levels.

Even though most men do consume the daily quota of 2.4 micrograms, statistics fail to tell the whole story. "We're seeing an increase in B12 deficiencies due to interactions with medications," says Katherine Tucker, Ph.D., director of a USDA program at Tufts University. The culprits: acid-blocking drugs, such as Prilosec, and the diabetes medication metformin.

You'll find B12 in lamb and salmon, but the most accessible source may be fortified cereals because the B12 in meat is bound to proteins, and your stomach must produce acid to release and absorb it.

A bowl of 100% B12-boosted cereal and milk every morning will do it for you even if you take the occasional acid-blocking medicine. However, if you pop Prilosec on a regular basis or are on metformin, talk to your doctor about tracking your B12 levels and possibly taking an additional supplement.

The vitamin B12 I take is in my multivitamins taken in the morning and evening. I also take a tablet in the evening about seven times a month to ensure my white blood count is within a healthy range.

Vitamin C Time Released (TR)

Years ago, I read where a group of chimpanzees were studied in the early 20th century by a German and, later, an American team of researchers. Their conclusions were almost identical. They observed that when these chimps were under stress, injured, or became sick, they resorted to eating more fruit, especially oranges.

Researchers found that what they were craving was the vitamin C in the fruit. If we, humans, tried the same, we'd have to eat crates of oranges as an equivalent according to this article. But, alas, with the advent of vitamin supplements, we can take high potency pills or capsules, instead.

Vitamin C is water soluble which means our body cannot store it for any great length of time. It just uses what's needed and passes off the rest in your urinary tract, unused. Within the last century, the time released (TR) version of "C" was developed and marketed to slow the absorption down. Thus, our bodies can more efficiently utilize this vitamin.

About 60% of adult men don't get enough vitamin C an *American Journal of Clinical Nutrition* study determined. It helps protect your cells from the tissue-damaging free radicals as a result of exercise. Vitamin C also helps heal wounds, and plays a major role in the production of collagen found in ligaments and tendons.

I read a long time ago, that when you take medication, it robs your body of vitamin C. I confirmed this claim with a sports medicine chiropractor, Dr. Bill Reilly of Houston, Tx in 2014. No additional research time has been taken to further validate this statement. Nevertheless, as a matter of habit whenever I take a med, I accompany it with 500 mg. of TR vitamin C. I rarely get sick which might be due to taking three doses of "C" a day plus the extra "C" I take when on a medication which includes an aspirin or ibuprofen. .

With the exception of a recent Houston flu epidemic, I've not been sick in many years. That includes flu seasons, getting a cold, or what have you. Notably though, when I'm in a new environment and a virus is active whose strain I've not been exposed to, I could be at risk. My resistance to viruses could very well be because of the vitamin C and other health habits I've practiced through the years.

Co-Enzyme Q10

Coenzyme Q-10 (CoQ-10) is a vitamin-like substance found throughout the body mainly in the heart, liver, kidney, and pancreas. It can lower blood pressure while raising SOD levels SOD is an enzyme believed to protect blood vessels from damage. Japanese researchers found CoQ10 can increase fat burning during exercise.

People use coenzyme Q-10 to treat heart and blood vessel conditions such as congestive heart failure (CHF), chest pain (angina), high blood pressure, and heart problems linked to certain cancer drugs. It is used for diabetes, gum disease (taken by mouth and applied directly to the gums), breast cancer, Huntington's disease, Parkinson's disease, muscular dystrophy, increasing exercise tolerance, chronic fatigue syndrome (CFS), and Lyme disease.

Some individuals believe coenzyme Q-10 might help increase energy because it plays a role in producing ATP (Adenosine-5'-triphosphate). In addition, CoQ10 has been used to treat disorders that limit energy production in the body cells (mitochondrial disorders), and improve exercise performance.

Additionally, CoQ10 has been used to strengthen the immune systems of those with HIV/AIDS, to treat male infertility, and migraine headaches.

Coenzyme Q-10 has been utilized with the belief that it increased human life span. Studies have shown that CoQ-10 levels are highest in the first 20 years of life. Conversely, in old age, levels were found to be lower than they were at birth. It was thought that restoring high levels of CoQ10 late in life might extend life. However, the idea works only in bacteria and not in lab rats. More research is needed to determine whether it works in humans.

Chromium-GTF (glucose tolerance factor) - **200 mcg**

Chromium is a metal and considered an "essential trace element" since very small amounts are necessary for human health. It is used to improve blood sugar control with pre-diabetes, diabetes Type 1and II, and high blood sugar due to steroid use.

Some active men take chromium for weight loss, to increase muscle, and decrease body fat. It's also used to improve athletic performance and increase energy.

Chromium might help to normalize blood sugar levels by improving the way our bodies use insulin.

GTF, glucose tolerance factor, chromium is the preformed chromium. Some people especially the elderly, may be unable to effectively convert the trivalent chromium to GTF in their bodies. Thus, chromium GTF is available.

Vitamin D – 10,000 IU

Vitamin D acts as a hormone to help bones absorb calcium. It has been linked to reduced levels of depression, lowered risk of colorectal cancer and decreased incidence of heart attacks.

The most common role for Vitamin D has been to strengthen bones. A study in the American Heart Association's *Circulation* found that people deficient in vitamin D were up to 80% more likely to suffer a heart attack or stroke. One reason for this was vitamin D may be responsible for reducing arterial inflammation. Thus, it reduces the chance of a stroke or heart attack.

Vitamin D is created in your body when the sun's ultraviolet B (UVB) rays penetrate your skin. The stored vitamin D from the sunnier months is often depleted by winter. This tendency holds true especially when you live in the northern part of the United States where UVB rays are less intense from November to the end of February. When Boston University researchers measured the vitamin D in young adults at the end of that specific winter, 36% were found to be deficient.

Confirm whether you've a deficiency with your doctor. "You need to be above 30 nanograms per milliliter," says Michael Holick, M.D., Ph.D., professor of medicine at Boston University. Take 1400 IU of vitamin D each day from a supplement or multivitamin when a deficiency has been determined. "It's about seven times the recommended daily intake for men, but it takes that much to boost blood levels of D", says Dr. Holick.

Recent research has linked low levels of vitamin D to obesity. For instance, in 2009, Shalamar Sibley, M.D. at the University of Minnesota tested the effects of calorie reduction on hormones and vitamin D. "Researchers have been tracking the relationship between low vitamin D and obesity," says Dr. Sibley. "So I wondered if people's baseline vitamin D levels would predict their ability to lose weight when cutting calories."

It seems that at the start of the study, people were likely to lose more weight when they had adequate vitamin D levels than those at lower dosages. Additional information about Dr. Sibley's work and other material can be accessed online using one of the available search engines.

DHEA – 25 micrograms after dinner
The DHEA hormone is naturally produced by the human body and can also be made in the laboratory. It's used to slow or reverse the aging process, improve thinking skills in older people, and slow the progress of Alzheimer's disease.

Athletes use DHEA to increase muscle mass, strength, and energy. It's also used for erectile dysfunction (ED) to improve well-being and sexuality. What's more, it's used for weight loss and to boost the immune system.

Be sure to read the labels and purchase this product from reputable sources. Like many supplements, DHEA quality control needs improvement. Some manufacturers whose products have claimed to contain DHEA in their product did not, while others contained more than the listed amount.

DHEA levels seem to go down as people age and they appear to decrease in people with conditions like depression. Some researchers think that replacing DHEA with supplements might prevent some diseases and conditions. I use it as a disease preventative and boost my immunity.

Ginkgo Biloba – In my multi-vitamin
Ginkgo is an herb whose leaves are generally used for medicine.

It's often used for memory disorders including Alzheimer's disease and conditions that seem to be due to reduced blood flow to the brain, especially in older people. These conditions include memory loss, headache, ringing in the ears, vertigo, difficulty concentrating, mood disturbances, and hearing disorders. Ginkgo is also used for thinking disorders related to Lyme disease and depression.

Some people use ginkgo to treat sexual performance problems. Ginkgo has been tried for eye problems including glaucoma, diabetic eye disease, and age-related macular degeneration (AMD). Little research has shown success in these areas.

Ginkgo biloba is one of the longest living tree species in the world living for as long as a thousand years. In fact, its use can be traced back to 2600 BC for asthma and bronchitis,

Ginkgo biloba seems to improve blood circulation which helps the brain, eyes, ears, and legs to function better. It may slow down Alzheimer's disease by interfering with changes affecting thinking.

In addition, Ginkgo contains substances that might kill bacteria and fungi that cause infection in the body.

This herb is in my over 50 multivitamin taken in the morning.

Multivitamin for Men Over 50
Since I've been over 50 for some time, I've been taking this performance formulated multivitamin for quite a while. It's part of my morning vitamin regimen. Designed for men over 50 years of age, it contains nutrients not commonly found in the diet or in other multivitamins like Glucosamine, Chondroitin, and Phosphatidylserine. Ginkgo Biloba, described above also helps with alertness and some memory issues associated with age. Also, there are elements in the formula to support prostate, reproductive and sexual health besides the ordinary B Vitamins, Vitamin B-6, B-12 and Folic Acid intended to work together to maintain cardiovascular function and homocysteine levels. Bear in mind that I've compared what it offers vs. a conventional multivitamin and found the additional ingredients are quite useful for the aging and active 50 plus year old man.

Multivitamin for Athletes
You may not need this multivitamin formulated specifically for athletes; it depends on your physical activity. Mine is extremely intense; I workout five to six days a week utilizing heavy resistance exercise or performing intervals on the bike/ treadmill. I take this multivitamin as part of my evening regimen.

The athlete-formulated formula includes a (branch-chained amino acid) BCAA blend which is very helpful in recovery. According to the reading material, the mix is designed for men of all ages who need a high potency multivitamin for hard driving athletes. It has vital vitamins and minerals needed to support energy production and nutrient metabolism, two critical factors for athletic performance and recovery. Also, I like the levels of antioxidants such as Vitamin C, E, and Selenium. Of benefit, too, is that there is Arginine in this multivitamin helpful in recovery and repair.

Protein

Most men eat animal products and we really do become what we eat. Our skin, bones, hair, and nails are composed of mostly protein. Animal products fuel the muscle-growing process called protein synthesis. That's why Rocky Balboa chugged his raw eggs before his early morning run; it was the protein. Since those days, nutrition scientists have conducted plenty of research. So, read up before you chow down.

By the way, most adults will benefit from eating more than the recommended daily intake of 56 grams says Donald Layman, Ph.D., a professor emeritus of nutrition at the University of Illinois. It goes beyond muscles, he says: Protein dulls hunger and can help prevent obesity, diabetes, and heart disease.

The question is, though, how much do you need? Check your body weight and be honest about your workout regimen or whether you've a sedentary lifestyle. According to Mark Tarnopolsky, M.D., Ph.D., who studies exercise and nutrition at McMaster University in Hamilton, Ontario, " ... highly trained athletes thrive on 0.77 gram of daily protein per pound of body weight. For a 180-pound man, that's 139 grams of protein every day." He goes on to say, ..." the only caveat for the older adult is that there may be RARE folks with renal failure (hypertension or diabetes as the most common) where eating > 0.77 g/pound could be deleterious. This is likely < 1 % of all older adults who are doing regular vigorous physical activity."

Those who work out five or more days a week for an hour or longer need 0.55 gms of protein per pound of body weight. Whereas, men who work out 3 to 5 days a week from 45 minutes to an hour need less, 0.45 gram per pound. That same 180-pound guy would need about 80 grams of protein a day.

If you're trying to lose weight, protein is still crucial. The fewer calories you consume, the more calories should come from protein, says Dr. Layman. You need to boost your protein intake to between 0.45 and 0.68 gram per pound to preserve calorie-burning muscle mass.

Many foods, including nuts and beans, can provide a good source for protein. But the best sources are dairy products, eggs, meat, and fish according to

Layman. Animal protein is a complete protein; it contains the 22 essential amino acids your body cannot synthesize on its own.

It's possible to build complete protein from plant-based foods by combining legumes, nuts, and grains at one meal or over the course of a day. But you'll need to consume 20 to 25 percent more plant-based protein to reap the benefits that animal-derived sources provide, says Dr. Tarnopolsky. Plus, beans and legumes have carbs that make it harder to lose weight. Besides, for me, it's a big pain in the rear to balance your diet using only plant-based foods. It'll take more time and effort to analyze and calculate. I spend enough of it watching the way I eat, already.

So if protein can help keep weight off, then, maybe a chicken wing dipped in a cheese dressing can be part of your diet. Not quite because total calories count, skinless chicken is best. You need to scale down your fat and carbohydrates. Look for a lean protein source such as eggs, low-fat milk, yogurt, lean meat, and fish.

At any given moment, even at rest, your body is breaking down and building protein according to Jeffrey Volek, PhD, RD, a nutrition and exercise researcher at the University of Connecticut.

There's one very important fact to remember. Most people eat the majority of their protein at their evening meal. That means you're fueling muscle growth for only a few hours a day and breaking down muscle the rest of the time, Layman says. Instead, you've got to spread out your protein intake.

Your body can process only so much protein at a single sitting. A recent study from the University of Texas found that consuming 90 grams of protein at one meal provides the same benefit as eating 30 grams. It's like a gas tank, says study author Douglas Paddon-Jones, Ph.D.: "There's only so much you can put in to maximize performance; the rest is spillover." It's like trying to put 20 gallons of gas in a 16 gallon tank. It's a waste of protein and money."

Eating protein at all three main meals plus snacking on protein foods two or three times a day like cheese, jerky, and milk will help you eat less overall. People who start the day with a protein-rich breakfast consume 200 fewer calories a day than those who chow down on a carb-heavy breakfast, like a jam-smeared bagel. Ending the day with a steak dinner doesn't have the same appetite-quenching effect, Layman says.

The added protein may help lower the stress hormone called cortisol, and that drop could boost metabolism following exercise, says study author Kyle

Hackney, C.S.C.S. "Consuming a protein shake during resistance training may speed fat loss and help build lean muscle," Hackney says. Further, "…fat loss is likely not subcutaneous fat, It's more associated with fat stores within the muscle (intramuscular fat) given the muscle cell will need a lot of energy to grow through pathways associated with muscle protein synthesis." People in the test experienced the desired benefit using 22 grams of protein mixed with 35 grams of carbohydrates. I maintain that you should still take in a whey protein drink with carbs right after a workout to ensure optimum nourishment and recovery.

To conclude, for the active man, eating about a gram of protein for every 2.2046 pounds (one kilogram) of body weight per day helps build muscle provided the protein is processed correctly. "A high-protein meal has a slight diuretic effect," says Steve Lischin, NASM-CPT. "This requires plenty of water." This "is due to the toxic effect that high protein diets have on the kidneys. Eating an average of 25 to 30 grams each meal is ideal," says Lischin. "Not only will you put less stress on your kidneys, but you'll also utilize more of the protein you're ingesting by giving your body only as much as it can use each time."

"However", Mr. Lischin adds, "We have seen lots of data in the last few years that show protein is a very overrated nutrient. It seems we just don't need as much as we've been told and in fact animal protein has shown links to cancer and other diseases (according to the China Study and other publications, including "The End of Illness" by David Agus). I believe the current recommendations have been influenced by lobbying organizations such as the American Beef Council, The American Dairy Council, The American Poultry Council, etc. It has been further promoted by supplement companies that have a vested interest in supporting the position that more protein is better. "*Protein* needs to be divided into five to six small meals spread throughout the day. Should you exceed what your body needs, it spills over unused as explained, previously; besides, it's a waste of money. One study, published in the *American Journal of Clinical Nutrition*, concluded that 20 grams was the best amount of post workout protein to maximize muscle growth. This study agrees with Volek's work.

Protein and Seniors
There have been studies that suggest men 60 and older need more protein than recommended for those younger. Just how much has yet to be determined.

Since I'm over the 60 mark, I take the maximum suggested amount described for the younger man. Until there is conclusive evidence, I intend to minimize my risk of taking too much at one sitting for the reasons already explained.

The September 2008 journal *Clinical Nutrition* noted that the elderly may need more than the Institute of Medicine recommended minimum of 0.8 grams of protein per kilogram of body weight every day. When seniors consume about 1.5 grams of protein per kilogram of body weight they may experience optimal health, muscle mass, strength and function (i.e., for a 150lb.senior, it would equal to 102 grams of protein each day).

Whey protein is a complete protein having an amino acid profile comparable in quality to meat, eggs and soy. The May 2011 issue of *American Journal of Clinical Nutrition* published a study that found taking just 20 grams of whey protein per day effectively stimulated muscle protein accretion. Noteworthy for the senior man and with regard to the prevention of sarcopenia, muscle protein amassment needs to be equal to or greater than protein breakdown.

The November 2000 issue of *Current Opinion in Clinical Nutrition and Metabolic Care* researchers from Canada's McMaster University noted that resistance exercise was an effective treatment for the muscle mass loss caused by aging. Researchers also noted that supplementing that training with amino acids, present in whey protein, could also help curtail muscle loss. Another study published in the August 2001 *Journal of Physiology* found that consuming 10gm of protein soon after (Soon was not defined in terms of minutes.) resistance training is particularly helpful with increasing muscle mass in elderly men. However, it was inclusive that taking whey protein without exercise would prevent sarcopenia.

My experience has clearly demonstrated that nothing prevents sarcopenia. Aerobic and anaerobic exercise will slow it down, but never stop it.

PABA (Para Amino Benzoic Acid) – 500 mg per day
This anti-oxidant helps in the formation of red blood cells. It acts as a coenzyme in the breakdown and utilization of protein. PABA protects against second hand smoke, ozone, and other air pollutants. It reduces inflammation caused by arthritis; improves flexibility and helps keep skin smooth. PABA has been used to prevent and reverse accumulation of abnormal fibrous tissue that occurs in various connective tissue diseases.

Resveratrol

Resveratrol is a member of a group of plant compounds called polyphenols thought to have antioxidant properties. It is believed to protect the body against damage linked to conditions like cancer and heart disease. Resveratrol is found in the skin of red grapes, but other sources include peanuts and berries.

Resveratrol has gained a lot of attention for its reported anti-aging and disease-combating benefits. Early research, mostly done in test tubes and animals suggests that resveratrol might help protect the body against a number of diseases, including heart disease, cancer, Alzheimer's disease, and diabetes:

➤ Helps reduce inflammation
➤ Prevents LDL "bad" cholesterol oxidation and makes platelets less likely to stick together to form clots that can lead to a heart attack or stroke.
➤ Thought to limit the spread of cancer cells and trigger the process of cancer cell death (apoptosis)
➤ May protect nerve cells from damage and the buildup of plaque that can lead to Alzheimer's
➤ Helps prevent insulin resistance, a condition in which the body becomes less sensitive to the effects of the blood sugar-lowering hormone, insulin. Insulin resistance is a precursor to diabetes.

Lab mice studies suggested that resveratrol might even help deter some effects of an unhealthy lifestyle which lead to increased longevity. Resveratrol-treated mice fed a high-calorie diet lived longer than similarly fed mice not given resveratrol. Resveratrol protected mice fed a high-calorie diet were spared from obesity-related health problems. This protection was thought to stem from resveratrol's ability to mimic the effects of caloric restriction.

Resveratrol has also been linked to the prevention of age-related problems such as heart disease and insulin resistance. Researchers believe that resveratrol activates the SIRT1 gene, a biological mechanism that seems to protect the body against the harmful effects of obesity and the diseases of aging.

Resveratrol has been shown to promote DNA repair in animals, enhance blood flow in human brains, and stop the growth of prostate and colon cancer cells.

Unfortunately, there have been few studies conducted in humans using resveratrol. Medical researchers cannot confirm the benefits nor do they know of the long term effects of its use by humans. Studies have not discovered severe side effects, thus far, even when taken in large doses. There may be some risk when taking resveratrol supplements. The product might negatively interact with blood thinners such as warfarin (Coumadin), and nonsteroidal anti-inflammatory medications like aspirin and ibuprofen by increasing the risk of bleeding.

Since resveratrol is unregulated by the FDA, it's uncertain whether the dosage consumers are getting is what the bottle contains. Furthermore, dosages vary from manufacturer to manufacturer. Another consideration is that there is not a specific recommended dosage to ensure product effectiveness.

Refer to Doctor Sinclair's research for more information found on the internet. His research continues and may produce a product for human use. Meanwhile, there needs to be better quality control to determine appropriate dosages and believable potencies labeled on resveratrol bottles sold.

My resveratrol supplementation comes from peanuts, grapes, berries, and red wines including the 20yr tawny ports. The red grape skin holds more of this chemical than the white grape. My daily (more like weekly) resveratrol dosage from wine isn't known. I'm not a drinker and I stay pretty close to the two six ounce glasses per day limit. There are more times than none when I just don't have much wine until the weekend on Sunday.

One final word about wine if you have to decide whether you want wine with your meal, order it. You just might protect yourself from dementia later in life. The Alcoholism, Clinical and Experimental Research from February, 2009 study suggests that older adult males who have two glasses of wine (or beer or highball) are less likely to develop dementia or experience a deterioration of age related cognitive reasoning than those who do not drink.

I offer one final piece of advice since I've been influenced by alcoholics in and outside my family. If you have an alcohol dependency, if there's a history of alcoholism in your family or amongst your friends, seriously consider another alternative other than alcohol to protect your brain from age-related decline. Heavy drinking can do damage to brain cells and serious harm to your liver.

Saw Palmetto

Saw palmetto is best known for decreasing symptoms of an enlarged prostate gland and does the work quite well. It's also used for treating certain types of prostate infections and is sometimes used in combination with other herbs to treat prostate cancer.

Some people, according to webmd.com, use it for colds and coughs, sore throat, asthma, chronic bronchitis, chronic pelvic pain syndrome, and migraine headaches. It's also used to increase urine flow, promote relaxation, and enhance sexual drive.

Saw palmetto doesn't shrink the overall size of the prostate. Instead, it's the inner lining that seems to shrink which puts pressure on the sphincter used to pass urine.

Fats

I thought it wise to talk a bit about olive oil touted for a long time as a good fat for good reason.

As a kid growing up in an Italian environment, olive oil was not only used for cooking, it was also part of our salad dressing. The flavor took getting used to, but I learned that real Italian salad dressing was made of olive oil and red wine vinegar unlike what grocery stores or restaurants offer as "Italian" dressing. Today, I use olive oil to cook and microwave food. I prefer balsamic on my salads which is closest to the authentic Italian salad dressing I had as a kid.

Olive oil is used to prevent heart attack and stroke, different cancers, arthritis as well as migraines. These are the claims, whether it works, I haven't a clue.

Nonetheless, studies seem to show the fatty acids in olive oil decrease cholesterol levels and have anti-inflammatory effects in humans. Olive leaf and olive oil might also lower blood pressure.

Water

Although, this liquid is not a supplement, it might seem to be one to those who drink mostly coffee, sodas, and beer. I've heard from childhood that we should drink eight to 10 glasses of water a day. Filtered tap water is my main beverage at home, but I do drink black coffee or green tea and enjoy a good full bodied red table wine. I, especially appreciate a good dessert wine like the 20yr tawny ports. I'll bet I drink over 100 ounces of water each day. How much or less depends on the temperature, humidity, whether I did an aerobic workout, and how much fluid I've lost through perspiration and activity during the day.

You can filter your water at home to minimize taking in any unnecessary impurities especially when you are undergoing mainstream cancer treatment and/or self-imposed healing anti-cancer alternative methods to be explained, later. Go online to purchase an inexpensive one like Zerowater.

The benefits of drinking tap water over other beverages are many. Water acts as an appetite suppressant which will reduce hunger pangs to a point; it's not all inclusive. It will flush by-products of fats during digestion. Through proper hydration, headaches and backaches can be relieved, believe it or don't. Water will help replenish and moisturize skin while making it more elastic. Drinking water can make you think more clearly and concentrate better. Water will also help regulate your body temperature. It will help in digestion and relieve constipation. Proper hydration will help lubricate your muscles, joints, and digestive tract as well.

When you drink adequate amounts of water, you can fight the effects of the flu and ailments like kidney stones and heart disease. Tap water has been known to flush out toxins and other waste products from the body. Studies have indicated that drinking sufficient water may reduce the risks associated with bladder and colon cancers.

The use of bottled water makes drinking water more convenient. It isn't the best choice, however, since tap water must pass federal, state, and local regulations. Although, bottled water is somewhat regulated, it does not have to meet these same standards. Moreover, natural minerals and anti-tooth decay ingredient like fluoride that tap water provides are removed through the bottled water cleansing/purification process. Thus, anyone who uses bottled water as their main supply may be more susceptible to tooth decay. You have to be careful of ingesting micro-plastics in bottled water, too.

Besides, tap water is free. Why pay for water that's less regulated and may have no fluoride just for the convenience? Instead, get an empty bottle and fill it with tap water if you're bent on bottling water. Make certain you avoid keeping bottled water or empty plastic bottles in your car for very long periods of time. When the inside of your car overheats, plastics can become toxic as a well-known female singer learned a few years ago.

Are you drinking enough water to effectively digest and assimilate protein by the body? It must be water not just another fluid in this instance. When protein is utilized for energy, it goes through a process to convert to glucose. Water and lots of it, is needed. A good deal of stress is placed on the kidneys when you drink anything else over water and they don't work nearly as hard to assimilate your protein.

Sleep
Schedule your sleep at the same time, consistently, for best results. You need 8 hours a night, plus or minus, depending on your lifestyle, how hard you work, how hard you work out, and whether you're getting good quality, uninterrupted sleep. Otherwise, you increase arterial aging and raise your risk of a heart attack. Inadequate sleep will also cause you to release less serotonin (the feel-good hormone) in your brain. Without good sleep, one might seek out other less unhealthy alternatives to feel good. There's bingeing on sugary foods like doughnuts or drinking too much coffee or alcohol. All this according to realage.com will raise your blood pressure.

An article dated October 12, 2015 on webMD.com entitled "*18 Secrets for a Longer Life*" says getting good quality adequate sleep can minimize risks associated with obesity, diabetes, heart disease, and mood disorders. Further, good sleep will help you recover from sickness faster. Conversely, staying up late isn't very good. When you sleep less than five hours a night you run the risk of dying sooner than later. And I've said good quality uninterrupted sleep is important for recovery & repair from the day's activities. Sleep should be a high priority for health and longevity.

When you binge, you'll put on the weight just because you didn't get enough shut-eye. The lack of sleep releases less serotonin in your brain which gives you the feeling of pleasure. To compensate, you try to increase those levels with foods like sugar or harmful substances like tobacco. Ignoring your need to sleep will only worsen things (Realage.com – All about You: What's Your Sleep Like?).

When you throw off your sleep schedule, your repair & rebuild cycle will suffer. To look and feel your best and youngest, studies show that men need to sleep a minimum of seven to eight solid hours a night. Why? You're body needs to recharge. Your brain, eyes, and willpower are depending on it.

Sleep is best when it's uninterrupted. The more uninterrupted sleep you get, the better, because that's when your body can benefit from rapid eye movement and slow-wave sleep patterns that are so restorative.
Doctors don't know exactly why, but if you get less sleep than you need, or you don't get enough quality sleep, it increases your arterial aging and the risk

of heart attack. Interestingly, not only do you need the proper time to sleep, but you need to clock solid hours of sleep. One major reason is that it takes about 2.5 hours of straight sleep before it becomes truly recuperative.

How much sleep is enough within the range described above? I believe so passionately about its importance some of the information on sleep bears underscoring.

"How much" depends on your lifestyle activities, tension, anxiety, whether you're sedentary or active, what you do in the gym. I can easily feel great the next day on seven & one-half to eight hours a night if I don't workout. My intense workouts require I get a minimum of nine hours per night otherwise, I haven't adequately recovered.

Over time, sleep deprivation is a silent killer. It shortens your life. The solution is to go to bed and wake up at set times every day, even on weekends, to keep your sleep cycles regulated. I didn't do that years ago and it's unfortunate I didn't have this advice at that time in my life. Also, you need to avoid caffeine and exercising too close to bedtime. Instead, it's better to have finished your training four to six hours before bedtime. Personal experience tells me elevating your heart rate before bed can interfere with good, quality sleep.

If you still don't believe getting a good night's rest is worth your time, then, listen to this! When fighting cancer or preventing recurrence, quality sleep is critical! Take the time to sleep; it's a matter of your life or death!

Anxiety/ Stress Management
Earlier in my life, I was a big worrier. In time, it changed when I gradually learned it was healthier to develop effective coping skills. Today, I refuse to clutter my mind with unnecessary worries like the "woulda-shoulda-coulda" game or agonize over issues I've no control. Yes, when I was younger, I was debt-ridden, constantly concerned about paying bills, and saving money. Those days are over.

Stress can make you sick, it's toxic. It's unhealthy for your heart; it will raise your blood pressure and you can lose sleep. All of this can impact your cognitive thinking. Stress hormones can seriously affect your memory; I can attest to it.

Part of effective disease management is handling anxiety and stress well enough to reduce emotional and physiological damage to yourself. One method I used to cut down on financial worries was to make a Want-Need List. What I "needed" had priority and it took discipline to plan before I bought. You read it correctly; I'd avoid buying on credit. In fact, there was a time I was so foolishly in debt, I had six credit cards to pay off. I got creative; I'd use one credit card to pay another card's monthly sum. It got old, never removed my anxiety about debt, and my debt wasn't going down.

Planning and restraint caused me to create a companion slogan-question: "Do I need it or do I just want it?" It was painful, but I learned how to say "No." to over-spending and I refused to listen to anyone trying to convince me it was "okay" to jack up my credit.

Rather than feel powerless over your dilemma, take control and don't let anyone including those close to you side track or talk you out of reducing your worries, especially, the financial ones,

There's more to anxiety and stress than just money worries. Much of how you manage yourself is based on what was learned during your developmental years: the guilt trips, insecurity, feelings of inadequacy, and how you reasoned matters challenging you at the moment. After a while, they become self-induced and, oft times, self-fulfilling prophesy. Sound familiar?

Stress does some crazy things. It can drive you to drink, overeat, smoke, or you can pick up other bad habits to try to cope. It's been known to kill. So, be wary, learn to effectively manage yourself. There're plenty of helpful internet sites to better cope and learn how to say "No!"

One good means to clear your head of personal issues is having a good physical outlet like exercise. There've been many times I've gone to the gym feeling upset about something at work or in my personal life. My high intensity would do most every time. When I left to go home, I had reached a calm I'd not have otherwise, achieved. It didn't mean I was over my worry; it was I had an outlet to constructively remove much of my anxiety and stress. Works every time!

I cannot see how people live life without a calming physical outlet to take the edge off what's bothering them.

While you're in this state of mind, your next challenge is learning how to put your worries aside before you hit the sheets. Otherwise, it will almost surely be a near sleepless night. I've had many such nights before I learned to stop emotionally beating myself up. I've been known to lay awake over thinking a worrisome event and how I'd handle it the next day. With few exceptions, my wasted time lying in bed thinking about such and such never happened the way I imagined it would the next day. Notice I said "the way I imagined it". My self-destructive thoughts kept me awake all night. I chose to do that to myself and if I can choose to do it, I can choose not to do it.

It's a matter of choice; take this worry to bed or leave it for the next day, you choose. Am I perfect, today? No, but I've had more restful nights than sleepless ones for years.

What about holding grudges? Do you have any? How many? Grudges especially unresolved, long term grudges significantly affect how much anxiety you'll endure for years. They become chronic anxiety!

Like grudges, there may have been times in your life stemming from childhood to the present when people have offended you. To worsen matters, you may have been, unconsciously, incapable of shaking off these feelings. They, too, will have an effect on how much anxiety you'll bear.

To alleviate them, have you ever considered the act of forgiveness? Letting go of these feelings has surprising physical health benefits. For instance, chronic anger is linked to heart disease, stroke, poorer lung health, and other problems according to webMD.com. Forgiveness will reduce anxiety, lower blood pressure, and help you breathe more easily. What's more, the rewards of forgiveness tend to go up as you get older.

Just how much anxiety you have will significantly determine the strength of your immune system. You want to do everything you can to maintain a robust immune system which will minimize the risks of acquiring disease including cancer.

How is this act achieved? Recently, I came across a method to relieve as much anxiety/stress as you're capable, all intended to strengthen your immune system. For best results, find a quiet time of your day when and where you will not be interrupted for at least 30 minutes.

Relax on your favorite sofa or chair. Sit or lie down; it only matters to you. Get comfortable; take in several deep breaths, relax. Allow yourself a period of calm for clear thinking and recall. Go back to an age when you first experienced feeling offended and when you held your first grudge. Think of these individuals by name and with heartfelt sincerity ask God to forgive them. Feel a lifting of tension from within. Once you've forgiven, ask God to

"Please bless them." Do this for everyone you can remember. For those whom you cannot recall, pray to God for these forgotten ones and forgive them in a general statement similar to "… for all those whose names I cannot remember, I forgive them." Then, follow this statement with your plea for God to bless them.

After this first "quiet time" session, you may remember others who've offended you or for whatever reason you begrudge them. Take whatever number of quiet times you need to forgive and bless these people.

The object is to reduce as much anxiety and stress to ensure you've the least amount of tension and your immune system is at its strongest. This method is an extremely powerful means to release chronic anxiety!

Each time I performed this act, I genuinely felt a lifting of pressure and tension never felt before these sessions. It works!

Developing useful coping skills will also extend your life. It all boils down to choices. How many guilt trips have you gone on this year? Have you yet to realize you've done it to yourself; it's healthier to acquire a more effective means to cope and you'll live longer for doing it.

To find what coping skill sets will work best for you, surf the net, take an online course, go to a half price bookstore, or take a night class. If all else fails, it's wise and healthy to speak to a therapist. I've sought professional intervention numerous times to successfully learn how to manage my stress. It takes a strong man to realize he cannot do it alone.

Studies Referencing Exercise

If you're not an exerciser, I don't expect to convert you. For the moment, though, before you decide to page forward to another section of the book, consider the studies below.

The University of Nebraska conducted a study on exercise involving 16 cancer survivor patients and resistance exercise for 12 weeks. Blood tests were taken before and after the program. The study concluded that resistance exercise produced more of the cancer preventing and fighting naïve T-immune cells in participants after the 12 week exercise program was completed than those who did no resistance exercise at all.

I interviewed the lead researcher of this study, Ms. Laura Bilek PhD, to obtain insightful information. Although, she couldn't explain why pumping iron produced more of the naive T-immune cells, she marveled at how beneficial they were as cancer preventers and fighters.

Findings of this study plus feedback from the MDA team assigned to my successful recovery validated my choice to weight train throughout my entire life.

There are many other independent studies that have reached similar conclusions regarding the benefits of aerobic and anaerobic exercise. Exercise reduces the risks associated with cancer. Dependent on age and physical condition, seriously consider starting an exercise program. You'll look and feel better with the confidence you're doing something to help your body fight and prevent disease.

What's more, according to the American Cancer Society, studies show that exercise is safe during cancer treatment and can improve many aspects of health including muscle strength, balance, fatigue, and depression. Physical activity after diagnosis is linked to living longer, plus, there's a reduced risk of cancer recurrence among people living with breast, colorectal, prostate, and ovarian cancer who exercise regularly.

For instance, a study published March, 2019 in *Medicine & Science in Sports & Exercise* states that older adults who lift weights are about 25% less likely to develop colon cancer than those who don't resistance exercise at all, These findings appear to validate prior research that purport there's a protective benefit to strength training and high intensity interval training (HIIT on cancer risk).

Previous research on the exercise habits of more than 80,000 adults found that those who pumped iron only twice a week were 31 percent less likely to die from cancer.

Also, HIIT might be a deterrent against colon cancer according to a study published in the *Physiology Society* earlier this year. Although, more research is needed, amazingly, colon cancer cell growth in colorectal cancer survivors was immediately reduced after just one session of HIIT.

Exercise
There's anaerobic and aerobic exercise and they, both, have benefits. In 2010, science finally concluded that the human body can remain active its entire life cycle. What's more, exercise reduces the effects of sarcopenia (muscle

atrophy due to age) that everyone experiences as we get older. Most forms of exercise will slow the process down, but not stop it.

Anaerobic exercise is comprised of any form of resistance exercise utilizing body weight; exercise bands; kettlebells; dumbbells; machines; or barbells. Studies indicate the most effective means of achieving success is to employ high intensity. Just how intense will depend on age and physical condition. Changing and mixing up your routines every six weeks work best to minimize the sensation of boredom using the same exercises.

Gyms, today, offer a variety of methods to resistance exercise via the equipment they have: kettlebells, dumbbells, barbells, and machines. The routine you select to tone and possible add lean mass will most assuredly depend on your desire, age, and physical condition. Depending on your experience at weight-bearing exercise, get a competent trainer. A lesser expensive choice is to surf the net for a trusted site that discusses resistance exercise for the novice to get acquainted with working out.

If you're over 40, I'd also recommend a helpful book "*Fit After 40*" written by yours truly offered on Amazon Kindle. It's an advice book covering topics useful for the newcomer/experienced exerciser: Aging; Lifestyle; Exercise Tips & Basics; How to Select a Trainer & Gym; and Exercise as We Age to name a few of the chapters. As you can see, this book is not an exercise book per se.

Aerobic exercise is for the heart and cardiovascular system. It's important to minimize risks associated with heart stroke after 50. Science has found with a rest heart rate below 70 bpm, the chance of heart stroke has been significantly reduced.

There's running and biking, where you do it is your preference. My choice is indoors in a temperature-humidity controlled environment. Whether I'm on a bike or treadmill, I know how fast I'm going and for how long.

Studies have shown that interval training is better than a sustained speed for a long period of time. I mix up my aerobics with a series of intervals and two or more Tabatas.

What's a Tabata? It can be achieved doing body weight squats, biking on a stationary bike or the treadmill. Warning: it's not for the faint at heart due to its intensity.

Tabata training was discovered by a Japanese scientist, Dr. Izumi Tabata, with a team of researchers from the National Institute of Fitness and Sports in Tokyo. It was primarily developed for the Japanese Olympic speed ice skating team in the 1990s. Each workout consists of four minutes: 20 seconds of high intensity work followed by 10 seconds of rest for eight sets. Dr. Tabata's team concluded high-intensity interval training had greater positive impact on aerobic and anaerobic systems. For more details, check it out online.

A word about attitude … Men need to view themselves differently with regard to exercise. Most of us, including me, have this sense of invincibility or macho arrogance that can interfere with making good, healthy choices. Realize men are not exempt from contracting cancer or any disease. Believe it or don't, disease prevention depends on how well you've managed your life with few exceptions explained later.

Meanwhile, whichever method you choose (Indoors/outdoors; bike/treadmill/jogging outside), you need to perform your aerobics up to a minimum of 30 minutes on your aerobic day. Those target minutes can be broken up into three 10 minute sessions on the same workout day as long as you achieve at least a total of 30 minutes.

I've been asked for many years, "What's the best exercise to do?" Although, it may sound like a cop out answer, "It's the exercise you *will* do!", several independent studies have reached the same conclusion. Exercise helps stave off disease including cancer. Whatever your choice, be certain you stay active.

Hormonal Balance
Remember I mentioned earlier in spite of my stellar lifestyle, I still contracted male breast cancer? One of two questions I asked before my surgery and treatment was "How did I get it?" There was silence; no one answered or seemed interested. Eye-contact was broken as all three medical professionals turned away. How unusual! I remarked to myself, "After all, this is a research facility and no one seemed interested in the root cause of my cancer?" To me, it would've been of utmost importance! More on this and my other question, later.

How I got this disease began when I was competing in bodybuilding on the national level while in my 40s. I'd taken oral and injectable steroids for just under three years (1983-1985) to compete against the other steroid heads. To be competitive, I, reluctantly, played the steroid game. At a five foot seven inch frame I weighed 185lbs; body fat was between 3-4 percent. As my doctor who supplied me with the 'roids said, I was going to "blow up" and I did; I was good sized for my height.

What did I accomplish while taking steroids? I placed in the top three in the National Physique Committee sanctioned Over 40 Mr. Texas physique competition two years in a row; won my division in the AAU sanctioned Over 40 Mr. Southwestern America (1985); and ranked in the top 10 of the country in the Over 40 Mr. America (1985). In all, I was nationally ranked four more times in those three years.

After I went off steroids and unknown to me, my system failed to naturally produce enough testosterone to adequately support a healthy adult male. I let this inadequacy slide for 23 years, abundant time for my body to become estrogen/estradiol dominant. Note that I'll be utilizing estrogen and estradiol interchangeably throughout the balance of this book. I began testosterone replacement therapy in 2008. But my extended hormonal imbalance, age, and getting back on "T" produced a lump behind the same areola as I experienced when in my teens. Nobody including me knew that my estrogen was past the upper limit for a healthy adult male allowing my hormonal imbalance to continue. Nobody knew because nobody thought of testing my estrogen level.

When this innocent appearing lump was diagnosed in 2011 as a benign tumor, I thought it would go away as it did so many years ago. Instead, I gave it sufficient time to become cancerous by feeding it every two weeks with "T" injections (via aromatase process).

As a point of interest, finding the root cause of my cancer was solely through my initiative with no assistance from anywhere include MDA. Mind you I researched the source of this cancer with no medical background. My conclusion was I created a chronic hormonal imbalance which resulted in contracting MBC.

Lesson learned; once a tumor of any size appears to be a harmless growth when it's first discovered, take heed! Remind yourself, you're not a teenage; you're much older and your body chemistry is different. See your PCP right away; get a biopsy to remove any doubt about what this growth suggests. Yes, it could be a benign gynecomastia. Nevertheless, if it's reasonable, determine the cause, then, have the damn thing taken out! Don't make my mistake! When hormonal imbalance is the reason, there are methods to correct it.

Following much research and numerous interviews with primary care physicians and MDAnderson Cancer Treatment Center medical professionals, I've developed a method that can reduce the number of annual male breast cancer cases when the cause is due to hormonal imbalance. Based on my presentations, these same medical professionals agree I may have found a means to reduce male exposure to this disease. Starting at age 50, I believe every man's annual physical should include a test for hormonal balance involving estrogen in the blood work.

Of the some 1200 to 2000 annual MBC cases in the United States, approximately $8 Billion is made by all the US-based cancer treatment facilities every year. What's more, about 450 of those men will die.

If I can cut those statistics in half, not only will more men live, there would be fewer annual MBC cases in this country. Although there could be a $4 Billion revenue loss by US cancer treatment centers from a reduction in MBC cases, these facilities could utilize this additional time to focus on other cancer cases.

I cannot emphasize the significance of hormonal balance between testosterone and estradiol to minimize risks associated with disease including cancer. When hormonal imbalance is determined, discuss with your doctor how balance can be returned.

Lifestyle
The manner in which you managed yourself coupled with your good and bad habits; whether you're active or sedentary all influenced how healthy you will be as you age. In fact, the above six descriptors, actually, are determined by lifestyle choices. MDAnderson and Dr. Mark Lewis have said one is more likely to contract any form of cancer based on lifestyle choices than family history. I go one step further. Excluding genes and age, one is likely get any kind of disease based on lifestyle choices throughout your entire life than family history.

Several years ago, a gym member I knew in his 60s approached me during one of our workouts. He asked whether I took meds for heart, blood pressure, or cholesterol. I answered, "No!" and asked, "Why would I be on prescription drugs when I can effectively manage them, myself? Besides, look how much money I save!" He momentarily stared at me in silence, shook his head sideways, and remarked "Awesome!" and walked away

.

I insist you can effectively manage yourself, save money, and live longer without prescribed drugs. It depends on genes and lifestyle choices. A big advantage of managing yourself without drugs is your liver; it won't have to work as hard vs. while on prescribed drugs, your liver would need to constantly detoxify your system. Another serious consideration is there are always going to be long term side effects being on meds for years on end.

Bear in mind, when I speak of lifestyle, the remaining six components listed will have a positive/negative affect on your lifestyle dependent on how you decide to manage your life; the choice is yours.

I've added additional sources relating to what professionals purport as good lifestyles:

- Dr. Stuart Nunnally: Biological Dentistry and Cancer Prevention – Discusses how he believes there's a connection between root canals and cancer and cancer prevention via how to effectively brush, etc.
- Dr. Rashid Buttar: The Cancer Conflict: Resolving the 5th Toxicity; focuses on positive achievement via resolution of conflict interfering with your successes. Remove the emotional/psychological toxins that impede with achievement and success!
- Dr. Ben Johnson: Stem Cells, Lasers, and Novel Approaches for Cancer – major lifestyle changes

Chapter
V
Controlling Estrogen/ Estradiol

General

There's very little published discussion about estradiol when it comes to men. After I was diagnosed with MBC, my initial blood work did not include how much estradiol was in my system. I believe it was an important missing part of the analysis and made sense to know how much was in my blood. In spite of MDA's partnership with the UT Cancer Research Center, there appeared to be no interest in how I contracted this disease. I always believed the information could be utilized to develop proactive methods to prevent future male breast cancer cases. Perhaps what's disclosed in this chapter will encourage further conversation.

Imbalance

Healthine.com and lifeextension.com says too much estradiol in your system will cause:

- Atherosclerosis, heart stroke, and coronary artery disease
- Infertility - Sperm levels in semen may fall leading to fertility issues.
- Gynecomastia – The development of larger male breasts or a benign mass behind the areola.
- Erectile dysfunction – Without a balance between testosterone and estrogen, sexual growth and development is impaired resulting in difficulty obtaining or maintaining an erection.
- Be at greater risk for other conditions; obesity, Type II diabetes, muscle loss, and breast cancer
- Prostate issues
- Heart disease, blood clotting
- Endometrial cancer when elevated levels of estradiol continue for long periods of time
- Feelings of depression, fatigue

According to renaland urologynews.com low estradiol will cause:

- Increased body fat
- Decreased sexual function (ED)
- Bone loss via osteopenia, osteoporosis.
- Hypogonadism per the *New England Journal of Medicine* (2013; 369:1011-1022).

Lastly, lifeextension.com warns an increase in mortality for men is significantly greater when their estrogen levels were either too low or too high. Similar references can, also, be found in the *Journal of the American Medical Association.*

In a study of over 3,000 men between 69 and 80 years of age, testosterone and estradiol serum levels were measured during a mean 4.5 year follow-up. Men with low "T" had a 65% greater all-cause mortality while men with low estradiol experienced 54% more deaths. Men with low estradiol and testosterone were nearly twice as likely to die (a 96% increase in mortality) compared to optimal ranges of 21-30pg/dL and 348-1197ng/mL for estradiol and "T", respectively. Further, this study of aged men corroborates prior published reports linking testosterone and/or estradiol imbalances with greater incidences of degenerative disease and death.

Balance
Under 60 Years of Age
A healthy estrogen range for this age group is 7.6-42.6pg/dL for an adult male. If during an annual examination, your blood work indicates estradiol was outside this range while your testosterone was in its healthy range of 348-1197ng/mL, hormones are out of balance.

60 Years of Age or Older
When your blood work during an annual examination shows estradiol is outside the range of 21-30pg/dL while testosterone was inside its healthy range, hormones are out of balance.

There're several ways estradiol can be blocked or reduced to its healthy range. Recognize estrogen blockers have unpopular and serious side effects. Thankfully, there are healthier, natural ways estradiol can be managed without the side effects blockers produce.

Prescribed Estrogen Blockers
Select the meds of interest, below, and surf the Net to obtain their side effects. Those medications that still remain of interest, discuss the pro-s & con-s of each product with your doctor.

If I had my way, I'd be strictly trying to reduce my estradiol using natural means and supplements than prescribed drugs. Furthermore, I would not recommend the use of estrogen blockers since they produce unhealthy side effects including death. Whether you will die from the use of blockers is dependent on your age, physical condition, blocker dosage, and length of time on the medication. Since, I'm under my oncologist's care and instruction; I don't dare go off my prescribed Tamoxifen. The good part is I don't have to take it every day, now, as I did the first three years. Dosage has been pulsed: one month on and one month off.

The use of the listed blockers is dependent on the cancer condition. As a point of interest, entirely blocking all of the estradiol creates a hormonal imbalance that MDAnderson does not seem concerned about; I've complained and they insist I must take the blocker than manage my estradiol utilizing a healthier alternative:

- Tamoxifen - Breast cancer treatment drug (Prescribed by MDAnderson)
  - Major side effects:
    - Sexual dysfunction: no libido
    - Weight gain: Usually an accumulation of belly fat
    - Hypogonadism
    - Long term/late side effect dependent on duration in years: death
    - Two less severe that I've experienced:
      - Hot flashes – some severe lasting more than five minutes
      - An odor in perspiration and urine
- Arimidex
  - Often prescribed in a low dosage of 0.5 mg twice a week to control aromatization
  - Know the side effects
  - Discuss other alternatives with your PCP.
- Letrozole
- Raloxifene

Natural Estradiol Reducers/Blockers
Not only does excess estradiol pose health risks, certain estrogen metabolites may promote hormone-related cancers. One method to reduce this threat is to include:
- A daily intake of *cruciferous vegetables* like broccoli, cauliflower, cabbage, Brussel sprouts
- Supplemental alternatives: Indole-3-carbinol and sulphoraphane - Check them out online
- Avoid soy and soy-based foods.

Our modern day world is guilty of producing an environment and products with estrogen-like chemicals called xenoestrogens that oft times pollute the foods and water we eat and drink. When we ingest these chemicals, the all familiar aromatization process converts them into estradiol, thus, boosting the estradiol levels in our blood. However, there are natural solutions to the problems of estrogen blockers, aromatase inhibitors (AIs), and estrogen detoxifiers according to heart-health-guide.com/aromatase-inhibitors:

- Chrysin (Dihydroxyisoflavone) – This blue passion flower flavonoid has shown to be the most powerful natural aromatase inhibitor
  - Classed as having a low rate of bioavailability (absorption)
  - Must consume this product with piperine from black pepper, dihydroxybergamottin (DHB) from grapefruit or both
- Button Mushrooms -Powerful aromatase inhibitor with good results
- Trans-Resveratrol –Weak aromatase inhibitor
- Daidzein (4'7-Dihydroxyisoflavone) is a strong isoflavonoid extracted primarily from Kudzu root
  - Not as strong as Chrysin, the body absorbs it much better
- Hesperetin - Created by metabolizing hesperidin in the stomach - found in citrus fruits especially orange
- Naringenin - Another citrus bioflavonoid whose metabolites inhibit aromatase enzyme and reduce estrogen
- Nettle Root - Contains the weakest of aromatase inhibitors
- Vitamin D - A natural aromatase inhibitor
- Turmeric – Known to help, by occupying estrogen receptors
- 7-MF (7-Methoxyflavone) – A natural compound with powerful aromatase inhibiting properties, superior bioavailability
  - Don't confuse this compound with methoxyISOflavone; 7-MF (It's completely different)

Not all compounds or supplements are listed. Additional online searching will be necessary dependent on your determination to reduce estrogen levels, naturally. Although phytoestrogens like Chrysin and Daidzein as well as natural SERMs (Selective Estrogen Receptor Modulators – breastcancer.org) like Turmeric and Resveratrol are primarily estrogen blockers, they may, also, obstruct some of the aromatase enzyme process. You will have to determine optimal dosages to ensure adequate use without undue illness.

Liver Detoxifiers
As we undergo the use of estrogen blockers and aromatase inhibitors, the liver's task to cleanse our blood becomes more significant. To help it effectively detoxify, these liver detoxifying herbs can be utilized. You'll have to determine dosages via online investigative work. Since I haven't used them, I cannot suggest how much to take:
- Milk Thistle
- Prunella Vulgaris

- Artichoke
- Dandelion
- Burdock
- Yellow dock
- Adaptogens
- Turmeric

Supplements directly affecting estrogen metabolism:

- Indole-3-Carbinol or I3C - Found in cruciferous vegetables
  - Works well with estrogen blockers.
- Diindolylmethane (DIM) – A metabolite of I3C
  - Strong and effective compound
  - Increases the amount of good estrogens while reducing bad estrogens and xenoestrogens
  - There will be a change in urine color while using DIM
    - Caused by toxins and estrogens flushed from the body
    - Best time to take DIM is before bedtime or shortly after you rise when hormone levels have increased during your sleep.

To be fair, use DIM with caution. Webmd.com explains that hormone-sensitive conditions identified with some MBC cases when utilizing the DIM supplement might worsen conditions due to its properties acting like estrogen. However, developing research also suggests that DIM might work against estrogen and could possibly be protective against hormone-dependent cancers.

Although, DIM is a recommended supplement, stay on the safe side before you use it when you have a hormone-sensitive condition (i.e., your "T" and estradiol are out of balance). Always, check with your doctor.

If you'd rather not take supplements to lower estrogen levels, adopt the following regimens as often as is reasonable:

- Eat white button mushrooms, citrus fruits, broccoli, brussel sprouts
- Spice up your food with turmeric and black pepper
- Drink a glass of red wine every day – Pinot Noir is richest in resveratrol
- Take a healthy dose of sunlight to increase your vitamin D levels.

Most men are concerned about body fat percent and losing weight which is directly related to how much estrogen is in your blood. Fat cells contain the aromatase enzyme and your level of activity (sedentary vs. very active). Losing weight and lowering fat percentage will help lower the aromatase enzyme and process. Detoxification, estrogen blockers, and aromatase inhibitors will help with weight loss says lifeextention.com.

According to *Life Extension* magazine, November, 2008, and May, 2010, as the man ages, his free "T" typically goes down to less than 15-20 pg/mL. When low free-Tis accompanied by an excess of estradiol (> 30 pg/mL), aromatase enzyme activity can accelerate. What's more, this excess activity will rob men of testosterone while their estradiol increases to higher, undesirable levels. This enzyme activity can be suppressed with absorbable forms of chrysin and/or lignans such as those extracted from the Norway spruce tree (HMRlignan™). When aromatase is properly suppressed, estradiol will be reduced to safe levels while free-T may increase since aromatase activity has been reduced.

As men age, a large percentage of estradiol is synthesized in abdominal adipose tissues better known as belly fat. A reduction in waist size will also lower estradiol levels. One method to reduce this abdominal fat is to restore the man's free testosterone to youthful levels. Nutrients that inhibit the aromatase enzyme can help boost these testosterone levels.
.

However, testicular testosterone production is on the decline as men get older. Thus, inhibiting aromatase might not sufficiently maintain testosterone levels due to the low naturally produced amount. A viable solution is testosterone replacement therapy (TRT) via injections. At today's prices, it's an inexpensive method, although there are other choices with a higher price: pill under your tongue, patch, or gel. To avoid the potential for aromatization, the use of a very low dose of an aromatase inhibitor should minimize this possibility. Refer to Life Extension's **Male Hormone Restoration Protocol** for additional estrogen-lowering strategies.

Whatever testosterone therapy is chosen, it becomes critical to the success of the treatment. A report by Dr. Stephen J. Winters entitled *Current Status of Testosterone Therapy in Men*, "the delivery of testosterone … in a way that approximates normal patterns and levels poses a therapeutic challenge." Thus, it's important to work closely with your PCP to track the effectiveness of the method and dosage when undergoing testosterone replacement therapy. Speak to your physician about alternative methods on the market.

What Do Studies Show?

There's a plethora of online information regarding unhealthy estradiol levels and their implications. Thus, refer to the following article relating to testosterone vs. estradiol: Gonadal Steroids and Body Composition, Strength, and Sexual Function in Men, N Engl J Med 2013; 369:1011-22.

Testosterone is the precursor hormone for estradiol produced by the aromatization of testosterone in the liver, fat and other cells. Nature created it for healthy bone density but its role in men's sex drive, body composition and other variables is a source of great debate. High estradiol blood levels can cause growth of breast tissue in men
http://www.excelmale.com/threads/442...ight=man+boobs

Numerous anti-aging/men's health clinics prescribe anastrozole, an estradiol blocker to men who begin testosterone replacement (TRT). Higher estradiol blood levels can cause breast tissue growth (gynecomastia) besides water retention (edema). Further, there is speculation that high estradiol can lead to erectile dysfunction, but there is no published scientific proof. Since higher testosterone blood levels can produce higher estradiol levels, the use of anastrozole will prevent breast tissue growth and erectile dysfunction by lowering any potential increase in estradiol. However, science has not determined how high too high is for this hormone in men. There's some speculation that low testosterone-to-estradiol ratios may be more closely correlated to gynecomastia and erectile problems than estradiol alone.

Bottom line, there's insufficient data to establish an optimal upper estradiol value limit. However, the lower end of this optimal range when estradiol is <10-20 pg/ml can lower bone density, increase fat mass especially in the abdomen, lower sexual drive and erectile function. If the prescription is to utilize anastrozole (Dosage range: 0.25 mg/week to 1 mg three times/week.) to lower high levels of estradiol, discuss the implications with your PCP.

Monitor estradiol levels after having been on TRT for 6-8 weeks to ensure appropriate estradiol levels are maintained. An ultrasensitive estradiol test must be used than a less costly method to accurately determine these levels and when anastrozole is needed.

The estradiol range in a healthy senior male ranges between 20-30 pg/ml. These levels typically do not vary until the man becomes elderly when they have a tendency to increase.

Conversely, extremely low to zero estradiol levels are associated with higher percentages of body fat, subcutaneous and intra-abdominal fat. Sexual desire and erectile function is significantly decreased. Bone density loss and hypogonadism has also been noted.

Reference material to confirm the negative effect of low estradiol levels on bone density: Relationship of Serum Sex Steroid Levels to Longitudinal Changes in Bone Density in Young Versus Elderly Men; *The Journal of Clinical Endocrinology & Metabolism* August 1, 2001 vol. 86 no. 83555-3561

More on Tamoxifen
Tamoxifen also known as Tamoxifen citrate is a commonly used drug to treat certain breast cancers in men. It blocks the effects of estrogen in the breast tissue and is also under study for the treatment of other cancers.

"While tamoxifen is effective in treating breast cancer in men, little is known about its toxicity," said <u>Sharon Giordano, M.D.</u>, associate professor of medicine in MD Anderson's Department of Breast Medical Oncology and senior author of the study. "This research will help doctors and patients better understand the side effects men experience. With this information, patients can make more informed decisions about treatment risks and benefits."

There's startling news about Tamoxifen: <u>https://www.cancer.org/cancer/cancer-causes/general-info/known-and-probable-human-carcinogens.html</u> Details of an analysis by the American Cancer Society reveals that Tamoxifen is carcinogenic in humans. For instance, it's been known to cause uterine cancer in women when taken for breast cancer. Although, men cannot get this form of cancer, they can very well be exposed to other types dependent on length of time prescribed, dosage, physical condition, and age. Furthermore, major side effects abound when taking an estrogen blocker over an extended period of time: heart issues, reduced bone density, loss of libido, hypogonadism, and death according to lifeextenion.com and cancer.gov.

Why would any cancer treatment facility prescribe a carcinogenic agent to their patients? How is this choice related to the strong influence of the pharmaceutical lobbyists/companies? Time needs to be taken to develop a safer drug with fewer side effects.

Male breast cancers are almost always hormone-receptor positive. Tamoxifen blocks the growth-promoting action of estrogen on cancer cells, and usually is prescribed for men after surgery and treatment.

MD Anderson is one of the nation's most active centers for male breast cancer treatment. Lead author <u>Naveen Pemmaraju, M.D.</u>, assistant professor in MD Anderson's <u>Department of Leukemia</u>, saw a number of male patients while working with Giordano. Professor Pemmaraju says men seem to experience different side effects than women, probably due to the differences in their hormonal makeup (i.e., Men have lower levels of estrogen and higher levels of "T" than woman.).

Tamoxifen Replacement?
Cancer.org has produced a list of carcinogenic drugs; Tamoxifen is on that list.

Dr. Ben Johnson MD, NMD, DO author/lecturer/researcher suggests Tamoxifen be replaced with a natural hormone called estriol. He has given his patients estriol for many years with success.

From what cancer.gov says and the success of Dr. Johnson, why not develop a drug from this natural hormone, estriol? It's the weakest of the three natural bioactive estrogens and appears to be safer for patients than Tamoxifen. MDA could partner with the UT Cancer Research Center to find an inexpensive, non-carcinogenic, natural estrogen blocker superior to Tamoxifen.

What's more, rather than block all male estrogens which would create an unhealthy condition, why not develop an algorithm for use when establishing optimal hormonal balance for each patient prescribed this drug? Realizing each patient's chemical makeup is different due to age, physical condition as well as other systemic differences. Such an algorithm would prove very useful and save calculation time.

This idea seems worthy of pursuit for the betterment of the patient.

Chapter
VI
The Start

General

Here's the gritty stuff in case you haven't been diagnosed with male breast cancer, yet! For your sake, if you were diagnosed, I hope you didn't wait very long like I did before seeking treatment.

I'm going to put you through what can be expected before, during and after treatment. Know from my experience it's not just a woman's disease. You've heard of nausea and fatigue? There are no pleasantries! I hope you never have to go through this ordeal!

My Condition at the Onset and Before

I recognize I'm far from the norm for a man is his 80s. Most men have chosen a softer, easier life of existence. They're typically sedentary, overweight, have osteoporosis, and, undoubtedly, on about six different medications because they couldn't survive on their own if they didn't take them. My life's been different; I've practiced sound health beliefs and effectively applied them since I was a teenager.

I've had plenty of time to practice what I know on myself, first, before I shared this wisdom with clients. Health and fitness has been a major part of my lifestyle; staying fit for such a long time has wonderful benefits.

I began resistance exercise at 15 to perform better as a high school three letter man (football, wrestling, and track). As I improved at resistance exercise I began competing in AAU sanctioned Olympic weightlifting, powerlifting, and physique competitions setting local and western NYS weightlifting records during my 35 years of competition. I was nationally ranked in all three of these iron sports for a grand total of nine times.

At age 52, I decided to stop competing; I'd had enough. So, I made a promise I'd maintain my fitness, aerobically and anaerobically, afterwards, for the rest of my life. Thus, I was extraordinarily fit going into cancer treatment.

However, the health of my emotional side took a bit longer than age 52. Like most projects I take on, this one would require more time, reading, and several therapists to get me through it all. It was never very difficult to remember I was extremely abused and in foster care from infancy on and off until I was 14 years old. There was alcoholism and drug use in my family: mother and half-sister. It took time to recognize and accept I needed to get emotionally healthy to effectively cope with life. By the time of my treatment, I was completely prepared to take on this disease.

My plan was to work my five to six day a week regimen as frequently as the treatment fatigue and nausea would allow.

Once Upon a Time

The start of the disease for me began unwittingly in 2008 with TRT; my system was not producing enough testosterone on its own. Getting cancer was in part due to my age; I was about to turn 69 and had no idea what effect long ago steroid use would have on my system. When I took steroids, I took big: injectables and orals. In less than two years' time, I blew up as I described earlier with a significant reduction in body fat. It was so low, I became easily chilled during the warmer months and had to use a blanket to stay warm when the a/c kicked in. After I stopped, my natural production of testosterone was never the same.

I went to a urologist for a checkup in my early 50s before my last competition; I was concerned about my libido. He advised I track my "T" if I wanted to correct my ED issues and maintain hormonal balance. Unfortunately, it took me until 2008 to take his advice some 17 years later. Talk about putting things off; I was the typical Macho-guy when it came to tracking hormones. "That's for women not men!", I exclaimed and believed that little blue pill to be marketed several years later would be answer enough for me.

As you'll recall, my "T" was way below the minimum level for a healthy adult male which caused an imbalance between my testosterone and estrogen. My body was estradiol dominant until my TRT began. Everything seemed fine for a while, except I felt a growth behind my left areola. I shrugged it off; no big deal! I had a similar one on the same side when I was a teenager and it went away.

Through my readings, I learned to ensure proper disease management, hormonal balance was paramount; mine was the converse. Estrogen had free rein until I got off my arrogant invincible rear end to begin testosterone injections.

But wait … this lump seemed to be growing very slowly. In fact, it reached a point if I accidently brushed that side of my chest or leaned against it while working out; it hurt, really hurt. I was surprised the first time I unintentionally grazed it during a workout. The pain was so intense, it traveled from the tip of my nipple all the way up to the base of my tongue. That son-of-a-gun-thing really hurt! I became acutely careful about that side of my chest knowing the consequence if I failed to comply.

Time Passes

It's the year 2010; like my PCP had said, I'd be handling heavier weights in my workouts while on TRT and I did. I figured, too, it was time to tell him of this relatively new resident behind my areola. He recommended I get it removed right away and gave me a referral. Since I was still traveling for my consulting practice, I put it off.

Now it was January of 2011; I still haven't taken the time to get this mass removed and it hadn't gone away. Instead, it continued to grow ever so slowly. It was time; I wanted to get it, at least, examined so I'd know what it was and whether I should sweat it. I went to a breast diagnostic clinic for sonogram and ultra-sound tests of both sides of my chest. A benign gynocomastia was diagnosed behind my left areola; nothing was detected on my right side. I was told I didn't have to return to the clinic. I failed to have biopsy taken which proved to be a big mistake!

Whew, no cancer! A smile engulfed my face ... I continued traveling for my practice feeling better and believing I could have this thing removed most any time, it didn't matter when.

The clinic's good news went to my head; I firmly believed things were going to be all right. I kept my PCP's referral information handy when I was ready to get the procedure done. Now, though, I was in no hurry. Making such an appointment for removal was put off, again. Nevertheless, I religiously checked this mass every single day. It got harder to tell whether it stopped growing.

What's more, I never knew leaving a benign gynocomastia alone and not having it removed increased my risk of breast cancer by tenfold. I ignored my PCP's advice convinced it would go away like it did when I was in my teens.

By late 2011, a new twist evolved. Now, it ulcerated just below my nipple with an intermittent watery, bloody substance. At the same time, this growth behind the areola seemed to be pushing outward as though my body was trying to naturally abort this lump. I would band aid it so it wouldn't stain my skivvy or outside shirts. I wondered what this bleeding meant! How much trouble was I getting myself into?

My ignorant faith insisted on believing this growth was a harmless benign tumor. Although I was concerned about the intermittent discharge, it didn't stop me from traveling to long distant projects. I was relying on what I had been told in early 2011: I didn't have to return to the breast diagnostic clinic and the mass was benign. Never did I want or even consider this tumor could become anything more serious!

I was getting scared; I returned to the diagnostic clinic in January, 2012 for another examination. After I signed in, I waited in the lobby. I was too jittery to sit for very long. When my name was called I stood up right away. I headed towards the sound of a male voice, a laboratory tech who shouted, "You don't have to come back …" I felt astounded he claimed I didn't have to come back when now there was an intermittent discharge.

His words were very clear! What? With a blank, disbelieving look I replied, "Yeah, but, now, it's bleeding!" The tech paused for what seemed an awkward few seconds and retorted the same message louder and succinctly. Yeah, right! I left the building hoping he was right, but the infrequent bleeding undeniably contradicted what I was told. Meanwhile, my nipple continued to discharge while I traveled throughout the country for my practice.

June, 2012, while on a project in western New York State, an unusual encounter occurred that reignited fears I'd cast aside. While casually strolling outside a shopping mall on a beautiful sunny Sunday afternoon, I spotted a handsome leashed Boxer with his "mom and dad" coming toward me. Without provocation, the dog came right up to me as though his sole mission that day was to specifically single me out from the crowd. He leaped onto his hind legs and placed his paws on my chest. He, then, began vigorously sniffing my left nipple area while nudging my chest with his head several times; he knew something inside was extraordinary. Whatever scent my chest was giving off, it must have been overwhelming! With a single strong exhale, the Boxer stepped back down to the pavement to rejoin his waiting owners. All three continued walking past me as though nothing had happened. Surprisingly, I felt no pain just shock. The incident ended there. It took a matter of a few seconds, but this dog had validated my suspicions. I was given notice that something wasn't right. I needed to see that referral!

As this incident unfolded, I remembered reading an article about an elderly woman's miniature dog who kept smelling and licking her right arm. She finally went to her doctor only to learn she had cancer. Her dog's persistent act saved her life. I believe to this day, that Boxer smelled something uniquely unusual inside me. As that possibility materialized, it scared me straight! I knew I had to get back home for the examination I've been putting off.

Diagnosis

Finally, July 2012, 18 months from my initial sonogram/ultra-sound diagnosis, I took the time to schedule an appointment with my doctor's referral. This damn annoying growth had to go! Meanwhile, I stubbornly clung onto the notion its removal alone would make me "normal", again. Once it was gone, then, I could move on with my life.

The day had come; I arrived early, filled out the new patient forms, and waited my turn. Young and old patients crowed the waiting room absent of the usual chatter in such a full room. I was a little apprehensive and embarrassed about the bandage; actually, I used two that day just to be sure I'd catch all the discharge. I casually checked my outside shirt; whew, none showing. Shortly thereafter, a nurse ushered me into one of the examination rooms. It was quiet, clean, and more confining than the waiting room. Time passed while I tried to keep an open mind, but I felt anxious hoping to avoid a panic attack. Eventually, the doctor came in, Asian. I've always had good experiences with Asians. He introduced himself, Dr. Yo   . As I removed my shirts, I apologetically explained the infrequent bleeding and reason for the bandages.

A little discharge proved my point as the bandages were taken off. Dr. Yo leaned forward to closely examine the left side of my chest. As he sat back up, I heard a very quick, resounding, "You have breast cancer!" It was too quick; those words resonated over and over in my head! I panicked! No, not me; I don't have breast cancer! I'm a man and men don't get breast cancer, only women do!

His declaration devastated me; my anxiety shot way up. I began to nervously pace as the doctor attempted to calm me down. He saw my condition as just a "speed bump" that could be treated. A friggin' speed bump? He saw it as just a speed bump when it could mean the end of my life? I quickened my stride as the doctor continued talking and following me with his head and eyes. I kept moving toward and, then, away from him. He wanted me to sit to talk this out. Not now, not for a moment; I was way past "calm down to sit and talk" for this day! I felt my blood pressure rise and heart pound harder than I've ever known it to pound. Was this it? Did I end, here? What about all the things I still had to do? Was I just to let them go? And what about me? What would happen to me?

Those chilling insensitive words absent of any kindness will always be remembered. I wanted to hear a sensitive, more sympathetic doctor talking to me. Where was the consideration for the patient? It was pretty cold and a tactless way to ease me into the truth, but the cold truth was out. I had cancer!

How could it be? I'd been healthy all my life with a great lifestyle and exercise regimen. Hey, I was no ill-informed flunky who has poor health habits! It was me, the indestructible, invincible John Bovaird he was talking about.

For the very first time, ever, I was distraught and absolutely scared for my life. Oh, I'd been in gang wars as a teenager and got scared, then, but, this time was different. I felt helplessly out of control. Change, once again, had a way of turning my life completely off course. What was I to do? How much time did I have? Did I have "everything" in order? Would I make it to this year's football season?

My mind worked overtime trying to sort debris from genuine concern. Now I've got to reapply my stress management techniques and develop a plan of action. What plan of action? There were so many questions cluttering my otherwise clear headed mind. Where do I start? I needed answers, right now, if not sooner! What more friggin' changes would I have to face? How long do I have? How serious was it? I better get my legal papers in order. What should I do with my cars? What about my investments? What about my beloved dog, Sophia? How would I tell Jamie and my sons?

All of this self-talk was going on in the background of my mind while the doctor talked to me. The conversation reached the point where he requested a biopsy of my skin and lump to validate his clinical examination. I calmed myself down long enough to complete the biopsy procedure, got dressed, scheduled another appointment for the following week, and returned to my apartment.

On the way there, my mind had time to begin racing, again, with more questions, things I had to do: things I shoulda-coulda-woulda done, sooner; and people I had to call. I waited too freakin' long! I should have had this damn thing taken out in 2010! I kept beating myself up about that shoulda, coulda crap over and over and over!
As scared as I was, I told Jamie about the examination and not so pleasant preliminary results. Her voice was somber and deliberate; I heard grave concern in her words. She didn't want me or Sophia to be alone and urged me to spend the night at her home. As shaken as I was, I welcomed the invitation.

I remember the call I made after I spoke to Jamie. Since my older son had been in medicine until his debilitating bone disease shortened his career, I called him. After a long pause and deep breath, I confessed that I had breast cancer. For the rarest of moments, he could hear deep concern and a never before heard seriousness in my voice. Still, John wouldn't believe me, became agitated, and expressed his displeasure over what appeared to be a bad joke. I insisted I wished I was joking, except this time I was telling the truth. For one of the fewest of times, silence replaced spontaneity and after a long pause, he asked, "Do you know the low percent of male breast cancer incidence? Do you know how rare it is for a man to get this disease?"

My son knew the statistics better than me; it was less than 1% of all annual cases in the United States. At that moment, I didn't know and sensed he could hear for the first time in his life an unsettling fear and unfamiliar tremor in my voice which caused him concern. His tone changed as he expressed his love. He wanted to know what I was going to do. I intended to wait for the pathology report at my next scheduled appointment one week from that day. He wanted me to call the moment anything changed.

I knew I was scared for my life; I didn't know what to think. I began repeating questions I'd already asked myself. "How much time do I have?" "Can I get past this?" "How do I face my mortality?" And so the monotonous questions continued without answers for the first time.

There was definitely one thing I knew; I was not going to be a victim and helplessly let things happen. It angered me and I was determined to learn as much about this disease as was reasonable. I intended to beat it IF I could!

After settling myself down, again, I called my other son, Marc. By nature, he's a perceptive man who can more openly display and express feelings. I got his VM and left a message; he was at work. It wasn't long before he called back. Although, he couldn't talk easily, he listened intently as I went over what I'd shared with his brother. A long silence followed before he spoke. Caught off guard, he faltered as he validated his love and pronounced his wish for me to be in good health. There was no doubt he, now, knew how grave my news caused him to feel. There was an unsteadiness in his voice as he continued his hope for me; I could sense he was about to cry. I disliked leaving him in this state, but I knew he was at work. I reassured him of my love and promised I'd call the moment anything had changed.

After that call, I spoke to a friend of mine, a widower who lost his wife to breast cancer in 2005. We met in November, 1995, at the gym where we worked out and quickly became friends. He, too, detected a change in my voice as I told my story. Talk about a solemn conversation; he immediately sympathized with me and hoped it was not as bad as his wife's experience.

Several deep breaths later, it was done. I did my deed, the news was told. Everyone important in my life knew as much as I did.

Although, I cannot remember the drive to Jamie's condominium; Sophia and I got there, safely. The trip took nearly an hour; I spent most that time muddling over my dilemma. What an extraordinary first night!

I relentlessly continued to over think my mortality. Ordinarily, television was a good diversion, but failed to hold my interest that night. Panic found me quickly rising from the couch often enough to make it quite uncomfortable for Jamie. I'd suddenly and abruptly stand up searching for answers; looking away, wall to wall for something that wasn't there, wondering and wondering. Then, I'd sit back down. Frequently, I'd leave the couch in a frenzied state ignorant of my direction to pace off my anxiety. The night wore on with no relief.

Bedtime was drawing near; I wondered how well I would sleep. The day exhausted me, but when I laid down to close my eyes for what seemed a short while, invariably wake up, wide-eyed, looking around in a panic. Then, I'd spring up to a sitting position on the edge of the bed to over-think the unknown. Except, it wasn't enough to sit, I had to get up, pace, walk and pace some more not knowing what room I'd reach a conscious awareness of my presence. All the while my chest was pounding; I could feel my ears pulsating. I have no idea how many times I got up. The fear for my life put me in auto-mode; my anxiety was way up!

Here I go with more questions and self-doubt, again! What do I do? What do I need to do? How about a will? Should I get "things" in order? What are my chances of surviving? All these questions and more kept interfering with what little calm I had left. For the first time in my life, I didn't have concrete answers or a way out! I prayed and prayed in a way I had not ever known before. I was literally praying for my life.

During the intervening moments in bed, all this interruption kept disturbing Jamie's sleep. She, finally, blurted out, "You've got to turn it over (to God)!!" That's when reality kicked in! I've used that very advice as an Al-Anon sponsor to help others overcome whatever challenges they had before them. Yet, I never thought of applying it, myself. I was obviously too close to what was going on. Nevertheless, I complied and fell into a deep sleep for the very first time only to be interrupted by the morning alarm. I was tired, felt ragged and spent.

I reluctantly started my day, the day after the biggest scare of my life. My blood pressure was causing my heart to pump in a way it had not known until now. Worry and anxiety plagued me in a new way. There was nothing sensational about my veracity; it was here and now, my reality. I feared the worst and kept trying to cope just knowing what I knew rather than what I imagined. Sometimes it worked and sometimes I'd fall back into my familiar self-made trap: running off to a conclusion that confused notion with fact.

I called my PCP's office to give him the news. With some hesitation in his voice, he assured me that I'd taken positive steps to find the extent of the damage; it was too early to know anything else until the pathology work was completed. My doctor (known as Dr. G) instructed me to maintain our communication like I had with my sons and Jamie. He wanted to be kept informed of any change.

It seemed as the days drew nearer to my next appointment, I was coping better although good, quality sleep was intermittent; it was improving.

The much-dreaded day had arrived; it was pathology report time! My air of arrogant invincibility and strength was gone; I'd been emotionally beaten. As I waited in the examination room, I became curious of the door Dr. Yo used to come in last week. I opened it to peer up and down a long hallway; I saw him coming with the report in his hand. After he glanced at it, he nervously swished the pages against his leg several times; doctors get anxious, too. He looked serious which didn't sit well with me. I quickly closed the door before he saw me and waited for his arrival.

Although, it didn't take long for Dr. Yo to enter, it seemed like hours before the door would open. With some hesitation, he shared the not so good news; the pathology report confirmed I had male breast cancer. He described his plan to help me recover from this disease should I decide to engage him. First, I wanted time to clearly think things over and get another opinion. Looking back, judging from what MDA put me through, Dr. Yo's plan seemed more reasonable.

Meanwhile, I wanted to find a way to get my blood pressure down! The pulsating thump inside my ears reminded me too often of what was still quite unclear.

I immediately called Jamie, my boys and widower-friend. In turn, Jamie shared my quandary with her relatives in North Carolina and Ohio. They're a very close family unlike mine. One of her nieces worked for a pathologist, Dr. John Sorge, who became interested in my case and wanted to speak with me.

The conversation went quite well. He could hear the fear and unsettling sound in my voice as we spoke. To help ease my discomfort, he offered questions I could raise with the surgeon who diagnosed me. He also extended a willingness to refer me to an MDAnderson (MDA) surgeon. I immediately requested a meeting.

The MDA surgeon's plan sounded well organized. After much thought and checking with friends and relatives, I decided to go with MDA over what Dr. Yo had planned.

Meetings were scheduled to meet the rest of my assigned MDA team designated to help in my recovery: a chemo–therapist and radiologist. I was told the three meet on Thursdays to discuss their action plans for each patient they've been assigned to treat including me.

Since our introduction, I've continued my association with Dr. Sorge. We've easily become friends and with it, I sensed a higher level of integrity in his professional opinions. I've bounced off questions I felt needed a trusted second opinion. When my treatment was over, Jamie and I intended to meet him when we visited her North Carolina families. It was exceedingly good having the confidence and allegiance of a quality individual like Dr. Sorge. His reputation, personal interest in my well-being, and friendship had made this experience extraordinarily more comforting.

For instance, he shared wisdom I'd imagined would come strictly from a guru. He posed one of the most profound questions I'd ever heard, "Don't you think all your years of hard training were preparing you for this moment, your biggest life challenge?" Astounded by the question, I thought for a long while before admitting my destiny must have been to prepare to work past my most harrowing, distressful life experience!

In the meantime, my MDA surgeon recommended another ultra-sound/sonogram and biopsy be performed. They were to help him develop an effective plan before he proceeded. While the technician discovered cancer cells in the underarm lymph node area during the procedure, she noticed how this discovery changed my demeanor; it wasn't good. How much more of the "not so good" news was I going to hear?

Surgery was scheduled for Wednesday, August 29th, 2012, my daughter's birthday (Happy birthday, Heather!). My last workout was the Monday before, aerobic day on the treadmill; four hard, intense intervals; rest speed 5.1 mph w/ work speeds up to 7.3 mph. I was especially looking forward to recording what I'd achieved that day in my training journal as a benchmark for the "afterwards" part of my recovery; assuming there was going to be a positive outcome.

Typically, I followed Monday's workout with the weekly start of resistance exercise on Tuesday (Split routine: pectorals, deltoids, & triceps). However, I skipped this workout to be completely rested for Wednesday's surgery since I was sleeping better.

Also, this particular Monday (two days before surgery), my sons and granddaughter came to help me prepare to move. My lease was up at the end of the month. Timing was good since Jamie and I decided to live together in her condominium. These three traveled close to 300 miles from the San Antonio area to give me a hand. What a relief and I was exceedingly grateful they'd come this distance to help! It was a big respite to see them eagerly do so much for their dad/grandpa John. The actual move was September 20th, but a lot had to be done beforehand.

What a surprise! My lovely granddaughter Lauren brought her boyfriend to help. I liked him, nice guy. His help was welcomed!

The plan was everyone including Lauren's boyfriend would stay at my home until after my surgery to help as needed. I was to stay at Jamie's. I was quite grateful they came! Their heartfelt caring will always be remembered. Sophia, my dog, was to stay with them.
  Except we're particularly close this is a first. She's never been away from me while staying in my apartment. Poor doggie; she couldn't understand why she wasn't going with me and how long I'd be gone. There was a never before discomfort in the background of her eyes. Both of us were going to feel our absence during this time, another trying difference and change to cope with.

Surgery
Wednesday, the day of my surgery arrived. I'd find out whether the cancer was contained and my fate. My surgical team was going to open me up to remove diseased cells from my otherwise healthy body. I was scared. Never

in my entire life did I have to worry about my health, the direction of my life, or whether I was going to even have a life. I had no idea if this event was a start of a new one or I was near the end. I reasoned I was only 73 years old and my health history was beyond reproach until this point. I was a living model of health for all those who knew me, an inspiration to those at the gym. Now, this boulder was being dropped on me.

After breakfast, Jamie and I headed to my home where everyone was waiting. Sophia was very happy to see me. There was no hiding it. Everybody could see the fear in my eyes. The air was somber; happy smiles quickly vanished after our greetings. Sophia did not have a good night. I could see her uneasiness; I hugged her close and kissed her to make both of us feel better.

As I looked at John, Marc, and Lauren, I saw unanswered questions, untold apprehension in their eyes. They came to me to offer assurances; their faces gave away their deep concern, having never confronted this experience with Dad/Grandpa John before. The moments ticked by; it was difficult to say anything upbeat knowing we all wondered what loomed on the other side of surgery.

It was especially hard for John and Marc to look my way without the start of tears forming in their eyes. Frequently, I'd see them quickly turn away to avoid eye contact. I embraced them: I'd known them all their lives, stayed with them all these years after we left their mother and now this? Here I go, again, with my free thinking imagination instead of staying in the present with what I knew. I had to stop acting on these self-destructive thoughts.

As a family, we needed something greater than usual. I assembled everyone to have a prayer circle for strength and to make amends. I was fearful of what lay in store for me and wanted to feel everyone's love at the same time. Important, too, was the opportunity I offered for any of us to settle what might have remained open between us. No one felt the need which filled me with gratitude and eased my mind. I encouraged all of us to muster as much spiritual strength necessary to overcome this ordeal. Everyone eagerly complied. We took turns sharing our own prayers out loud which seemed to ease any remaining anguish. I assured everyone I loved them and didn't wish to leave them.

Time was getting shorter; we had less than an hour to leave. No one really knew what to say. An awkward quietness lingered while the minutes ticked away. Marc was sitting in my business office chair staring at the wall while tapping his fingers. Lauren uncomfortably tried to find something to do. John made himself busy looking for holes from wall hangings to fill in. Jamie was her reserved self just waiting, silently.

The time finally had come to leave; I kissed my beloved Sophia "Goodbye!" She didn't understand why she had to stay behind. I'd just returned a short while; I assured her I'd be back. Marc stayed with her until he was relieved by his brother. He and I embraced in a wholesome father-son type, the kind you'd see in movies after a long absence. We didn't let go right away knowing we were treading in the unknown. Marc is such a wonderful, caring son!

Whatever fate awaited me was a short three miles away. The ride to the hospital proved a quiet one; hardly anyone spoke. Helplessness was in the air as we absorbed its toxicity; what lay ahead was new. I kept thinking, "This, too, shall pass!"

After Admissions and prelims, I was wheel-chaired to my room where we waited some more. I had to change into those unmanly gowns that stayed open in the back. Surgery was planned for the afternoon; we got there early as instructed. Was my surgery going to be on time or was I going to have to wait?

Lucky me, it was delayed two friggin' hours! The postponement created a flurry of anxiety, anticipation, and, of course, my anesthesia worries returned. Looks like I'd have to stay overnight for observation, too. I was as upbeat as I could be, joking around with my family who took me more on the serious side. They politely smiled at what ordinarily would have been laughable, except not today. Jamie was prepared to stay over. Goody, maybe a PJ party with favors and ice cream later on? Probably not!

Meanwhile, everyone was growing impatient. As I lay on the gurney, I couldn't remember when the left side of my chest was prepped, but it was cleared of all manly hair, chest, underarm, and forearm. A nurse came to give me an injection that was supposed to calm me. It must have worked; much of my anxiety had left me.

After what seemed an eternity, the man dressed in white came to announce it was "my turn". My family wished me well and touched me as I was wheeled past them. Their looks told me how gravely worried they were for me like they thought nobody could see the way they looked. Jamie followed; she was extraordinarily quiet. I offered her a lift, but she declined. Not knowing what was on the other side, I chose to lightly banter a bit. The hallway was crowded with the typical masses focused on their private missions whatever they were. I nervously did my honk like a squeeze horn; people cleared the way as we passed not knowing where the horn sound came from. We halted in front of Surgery. Jamie kissed me and turned away before we proceeded inside. I wondered whether I'd see everyone after this part of my journey was over; I knew my body would never be same again. Maybe this was the end of my story ...

I was transferred onto the operating table; IVs were put in my right arm. For the life of me I cannot remember when my left side was painted "this side". Maybe it was after I was given the sedative. A nurse leaned over to instruct me I'd be going to sleep. Music was playing in the background, ZZ-Top, but I couldn't remember the group's name. Before I could finish my question to the nurse, I was rudely awakened in recovery; surgery was over. What!? That soon?

As I was wheeled back into my room, my entire entourage was there to greet me. What a wonderful feeling to see everybody! I closely scrutinized what surgery had done; I was never to be whole, again. Sure enough, my left arm was a bit impaired. There were two draining tubes coming out of my ribcage under my arm, the result of the removal of lymph nodes I'm told. And, boy was I ever thirsty! I drank and drank water which meant I spent a lot of time emptying my bladder all night long.

A single lumen PowerPort device had been permanently implanted under my skin in my upper right chest region for chemo infusions. It led down to one of my main heart arteries. Oh, goodie! After my cancer treatment was finished, I'd been told it will be removed by way of a simple out-patient procedure.

I took another peek inside my gown ... My chest was quite different, no more chest-posing for me. I was missing the left areola (nipple), that damn tumor, breast tissue, diseased skin, and an unknown number of lymph nodes underneath my armpit. I couldn't quite see how large my scars were going to look. Those two catheters dangling on my left side were intended to drain fluids from the lymph node area into medium sized reservoirs. The left side of my chest felt very tight. No doubt it was from the removal of skin and re-suturing what was left of me to close me up. I suspect I'll have quite a large scar.

Inconsequential at this time, but I had some overthinking to do. I became concerned about how that infusion line was going to affect my lifestyle and workouts. Or was it how I was going to modify my lifestyle and working out while wearing this infusion line?

Like I figured, I had to stay overnight for observation and Jamie was right there with me all the way. She's an amazing woman; I've never known anyone else like her! What a thing for her to go through and she's right there, nary a flinch! Never has any other woman been so sacrificial!

I thought about the pathology report that still had yet to be issued. It would tell me and the doctors where I stood. All I knew was my family was told the surgery went well. Good, except I wanted to know the details of that report. I wish I knew my BP count and heart rate right now.

Close to mid-day the next morning, I was released after my mandatory bowel movement. That was fun, but I "got 'er done" and we were on our way home.

Pathology
At my first post-op appointment the pathology report was discussed with my surgeon. Nine lymph nodes were removed along with skin, the tumor, and areola. The entire debris taken weighed about 11 ounces. A closer examination of the lymph nodes revealed, they were cancerous, but their margins were clean suggesting the cancer was contained and had not metastasized. It all sounded good and "good" is what I needed to hear. A scheduled CT (computerized tomography) scan in early September would confirm whether any other cancer cells could be found in me.

What an experience! I'd lost 14lbs, dropping down to nearly 165lbs. My clothes fit loosely which made me self-conscious; I was always proud of the way I dressed. My weight loss and temporary break from training was a setback, one I intended to get behind me, quickly.

The left side of my chest had significantly changed; it would never look or be the same, again. Acceptance was paramount. The remaining skin on that side took until 2016 to begin to feel normal like the right side. And the scar? It's a long one from the front of my left chest to underneath my left armpit-ribcage area. All the "bad" parts were gone never to impact my health, again. The surgeon had done a commendable job!

What's more, I had an added temporary task. These dangling tubes with reservoirs must be emptied daily; they're quite annoying and cumbersome. I was expected to record the amount of fluid lost. IF I met a certain undisclosed criteria by a specific date, I could have them removed and that side sutured. What a freakin' pain to have them dangling under my shirts!

Well, I survived surgery and pathology issued promising news. I'm expected to wait a bit to move on to my next wonderful recovery experience whatever the heck that was supposed to be …

Chapter
VII
Post-Surgery

General

The good news was no more surgery and things were looking better, but it's only the beginning of my MBC cancer treatment journey. .

My hope is you'll never have to put your family, friends, and yourself through the anxiety, fears, anguish, and challenges after having been diagnosed with breast cancer. Better, yet, I hope you don't have MBC and are reading this book to prevent acquiring the disease.

Whatever your motive, take heed to avoid my mistakes; know, first hand, what I went through to impress upon you it's no fun! What's more, there's much you can do to avoid/prevent this disease, altogether.

About a week following surgery, I met with my surgeon to discuss MDA's plan and have him examine his work on my chest. My cancer treatment was to be a simple, but lengthy process, a total of nearly nine months from the day of surgery to the last day of radiation. I was to have two phases of chemotherapy; the first one was scheduled to start October 1st. This phase consisted of a one chemical (Taxol) infusion once a week for 12 weeks. Then, I was to be subjected to three different chemicals referred to as FAC once every three weeks, four consecutive times. Radiation was next requiring 30 minute sessions, five days a week for six weeks. What worried me was the potential damage to my left lung and heart. I wanted to avoid permanent damage to any body organs, but was I dreaming?

After the chemo and radiation was through, I'll have to take an anti –estrogen pill every day for five years. To me, it was another pill to add to my repertoire of daily pills that supplemented my diet. No big deal until I found out the side effects.

Big on my list was how permanent any side effects, "late" effects, and organ damage was I to expect. This was an opportune time for my surgeon to corroborate such fears or disclose what I might potentially expect/experience, but, strangely, nothing was said. Furthermore, according to my oncologist, there was little risk with post-surgery treatment. Conversely, if I refused treatment, I'd have a 60-65% chance of the same cancer recurring. By deciding to take the treatment, I could lower the recurrence percentage to about half, in the 35% range. The chance of permanent organ damage was determined to be less than 1%, about 0.6% or a little higher. The numbers were persuasive and indisputable; I decided to undergo the treatment. Secondary to all of this was the inherited lymph-edema in my left arm and left side of my chest from the removal of nine lymph nodes. I'll always have this fluid build-up and have to go to MDA physio-therapy to learn how to mechanically move the fluid away from that part of my body. I'm expected to wear a compression sleeve to assist in fluid reduction. This daily routine would have to be done for the rest of my life. Welcome to the wonderful fringe benefits of male breast cancer!

It's Complicated

Timing is everything; I had a lot of planned things going on which became more problematic after surgery, catheters, and any temporary limitations. For one, I'd given notice to move out of my apartment after having lived there 17 years. I liked it there with my own private garage, the clean air, palm trees, being near the Gulf, the restaurants, and I was across from the Johnson Space Center. Too, I'll miss an AA-Al-Anon recovery facility where I regained my freedom from influence by someone else's drinking; I was plagued by that dysfunction since childhood. Next, my 14 year old dog, Sophia, had to have her tummy tapped every week due to fluid build-up brought on by her congestive heart condition. Lastly, I was preparing to move into my finance's condominium by September 30th and needed to get more boxes to pack. I was giving up a lot and gaining much.

Now, post-surgery and those dangling tubes have a way of interfering with my long time independence. It was hard to reach out to my sons for help. I needed to be certain all I've planned was finished by the time I was ready to move. I know I'll have a limited range of motion on my left side for a while. I had to get the big stuff done before surgery: the touch-up painting, filling in holes from picture frames, taking things to Goodwill, packing much of the big items, and having the Salvation Army pick up artifacts I'll no longer need.

More Testing

Shortly after surgery, a blood sample was taken for breast cancer susceptibility genetic testing called BRCA Analysis 1 & 2. It's used to determine whether I had been pre-programmed for breast cancer or any other cancer types, and if I've passed this gene onto my children.

More good news, test results revealed nothing pre-programmed me for this ordeal nor would I be passing anything onto my children. Even better news, the BRCA2 test results indicated I had no muted genes, either,

Later in September, I met with my chemotherapist who had already suspected the cancer had not spread based on clinical examinations and my behavior. He wanted to confirm his clinical evaluations and ordered scans of my chest, abdomen, pelvis, and bone.

More terrific news … The scans showed all those areas were clean. We caught this life-changing disease in time; surgery had removed all the cancer before it metastasized. I've something less to worry about in my recovery. I wondered though, how much risk existed that a micro-cancer cell had passed by, undetected.

The day before my first chemo infusion slated for October first, I had to sign a consent form. An MDA Administrative employee, brought it to me while I waited in an office-like area of MDAnderson. Get this! I specifically asked "Was there anything I needed to know about the treatment before I sign?" Silence accompanied by a big smile quietly urging me to sign was her reply. This was an opportune time for MDA to disclose what I could expect. Instead, nothing was said about side or "late" effects or permanent organ damage. After what seemed a long awkward moment of more silence, I cratered and signed without demanding an answer. Was this a prelude to other similar moments?

Years later, I sought legal advice and was told I could do nothing, legally, which seemed criminal and absurd!

Reactivation
Now, for the highly extraordinary experience I went through as chemo infusions advanced into the weeks ahead. What I'd experienced will be of immense benefit for those who know little of chemical therapy.

While staying at my finance's home following surgery, I took advantage of her exercise equipment. She had a treadmill and some adjustable dumbbells. They were light, but I reasoned it was wiser to take it easy on myself for a while. With all the orthopedic surgeries I've had and rehabilitation that followed during my competition years, I was quite familiar with exercising prudence during recovery. Although, this surgery was different, rehab should be similar. Atrophy was a concern as was sarcopenia at this advanced age. It's common for surgically affected muscle to quickly atrophy after surgery.

My first workout was five days after surgery. I was on the treadmill the afternoon of Septembe3rd. Since I had two catheter reservoirs dangling on me, I knew I had to be extra careful. I chose to stay at a low walking speed of 3.5mph and elevate the treadmill instead of increasing mph.

I, also, had to consider the port permanently planted in my chest. It fed into a main artery leading to my heart. I questioned its effect on my breathing, oxygen to my heart, endurance, and resistance training. It was all new and another change I was forced to maintain vigilance over.

I developed an intervals' workout comprised of a rest elevation for two minutes and a work elevation for one minute. The speed remained constant at 3.5mph. I started low to see how the catheters' behaved. My T-shirt seemed to have them comfortably against me to control their movement. There were 15 elevations on this treadmill. I cautiously chose work level 5 and planned to increase two levels every time I completed that interval. My purpose was an increased heart rate for a sustained period utilizing the interval training principle. The idea worked well and I was on my way back to some kind of fitness.

My first resistance workout was the next day. A serious consideration was my left side, the surgery site. Although, my arm was not in a sling, I had to be careful. My chest and latissimus area was sutured, plus, those reservoirs were hanging and draining from tubes between my ribs. Since I was unable to raise my arm overhead just yet, I had to improvise. I used leverage and the doorway to do limited range dumbbell side laterals. This exercise was followed by limited range of motion pushups and tricep pushups. I felt pretty good, after my endorphins kicked in.

Wednesday was core aerobic day. It went well as long as I stayed conscious of my limitations and medical apparatus on/in me.

Thursday was leg day and another time to improvise. With my limited abilities due to the port and catheters, I decided on single legged dumbbell squats, standing single leg dumbbell toe raises and high rep dumbbell hamstring deadlifts. It was a good workout.

Friday focused on lats, rear delts, and biceps as reasonably as my condition would permit. I used light dumbbells where appropriate in combination with my red exercise band. The workout went well.

These interim workouts continued until I felt ready to return to the gym and the catheters were removed.

Back to Normal?
As my chemo-therapy progressed, so did the physical change within and outside me. In fact, I was back in the gym the very day I started my infusions (juicing as I called it), October 1st. It was exactly one month and three days after surgery.

I was enthusiastic about hitting the heavier weights and seeing my gym friends, again. It felt good to be back. There was a lot I had to work on: range of motion, form, strength, and endurance. As each weekly juicing passed, change emerged in my awareness, drive, stability, and focus. Some say I had lost color in my face; I was less apt to crack a joke or laugh. The smile that was so freely displayed had gone.

My first six weeks of working out concentrated on basic muscle groups of the chest, lower back, and legs. Workouts were complete in the sense I exercised all muscle groups as planned in my routine. I focused on basic exercises designed to stimulate growth: benches, deadlifts, and squats. Using prudence, I relied on machines to compensate for my limited range of motion brought on by surgery. Eventually, the all familiar endorphin rush I'd missed, returned. I welcomed it back like a friend.

My game plan worked; I regained half of the lean mass I'd lost. At the same time, though, the chemo was getting to me. During my core aerobics, I came to realize I'd lost endurance. Ordinarily, I'd do three or four rounds with no rest. Now, I had to catch my breath at the end of each round which was a big difference from my norm! Treadmill intervals had to be significantly reduced. Refer to my *Phase One Side Effects* section for details.

By about the third week of chemo, everything changed, again. The nausea and fatigue grew on me. I bought an over the counter anti-nausea liquid to quiet down my stomach. It worked and seemed to raise my energy. My great and wise chemo-therapist cautioned that I'd eventually have to take a prescribed anti-nausea medicine for chemo patients. I scoffed at the idea, not me.

I also noticed my taste for meat had changed. Where I previously enjoyed seafood, poultry, or buffalo meat, not now! Just to be near them or pick up their scent from another room made me nauseous. More wonderful change!

Then, it happened … starting just before chemo infusion week nine. I had the worst 10 days I'd experienced in my life. Literally no energy remained after the infused steroid wore off and nausea as bad as I'd ever felt overwhelmed me! I'd hit a wall and there was no getting through it.

My oncologist would typically meet with me before each infusion to discuss my progress and Complete Blood Count (CBC) numbers. This time I had a confession; the treatment had finally worn me down to submission. I was unable to physically continue my core aerobic day workout without stopping before its completion. Exhaustion set in at the tail end of my first of four planned rounds. I couldn't go on without rest; the fatigue was too great to endure. Dr. Kovitz looked at me in amazement saying, "You've gone through several weeks of chemo!" He was astounded that I reached this far in my treatment without succumbing to the chemo-induced fatigue during my highly intense activity. He advised I go easier on myself; take more frequent rest breaks and remain vigilant of the chemical burden on my system. After all, I was under treatment that few could endure without fully collapsing from normal activity let alone intense physical exercise.

Funny thing, too, the chemo was not enough to cause vomiting, feel faint or pass out; I teetered on the edge without falling. The nausea and fatigue lingered long enough for me to feel miserable and lose interest in food, altogether. Everything I did that week was achieved with extreme determination. Even lifting my arms took more effort and thought than I'd ever imagined. No matter what I did, I had to lie down and nap for several hours afterward. Surprisingly, I still worked out and did whatever else I expected to do to carry on with life. No matter the task, sleep was a must after each undertaking.

During this time, commonplace tasks or simple everyday activities became a test of endurance. The nausea and excruciating fatigue caused me to think and over think everything. My body didn't want to work. I had to do my errands. The nightmarish detail of what had to be done to get through the day overwhelmingly cluttered my mind. Each and every minute detail was laid out whether I wanted to deliberate or not. For whatever reason, I had to ensure what I did was completed with the highest expectations in my mind, first. Workouts proved the biggest challenge. First, I became acutely aware of the elemental steps it entailed to get to the gym, complete my workout and get back home. It took everything I had to carry out successfully each phase, each detail to finally see the finish line. I was literally conscious of every incremental action necessary to pack my training bag; change into my gym clothes; take my protein drink; leave the condo; and so on and on to make it to the gym. Then, it was the same monotony in reverse to safely get back home. I'd leave the gym intently conscious of all the laborious detail needed to travel that 4.7 mile stretch back to the condo near collapse before I could take another rest. But, first, I had to park, turn off the engine, get out, get my gym bag from the trunk, lock the car, walk around the car to climb the 16 steps to reach the condominium door to unlock it, step inside, and so on and so on and on and on in my head. The minute, fundamental detail of it all jam-packed my psyche. For some contradictory reason, I was compelled to over-think everything, every step before I could act on it. It was nightmarish in a dream I was actually living for these several days. I could "feel" my mind working and over-working while refusing to let go of the monotonous detail of my daily activities.

Of all these major developments, my aerobic days became the most demanding. Doing anything for a sustained intense duration genuinely exhausted me to a level I'd never reached before chemo. Utilizing an interval training tempo from a rest speed to work speed was most challenging. Although I was spent, I never passed out or collapsed. Energy had left me to dwell on what I had once believed to be an out of place question ... how worthy was my unwavering quest to complete this workout? Rest became a highly appreciated time to recuperate and genuinely feel revitalized. I could bask in this lull. That's when I realized I had no endurance. The chemo had drained me. I reluctantly surrendered to its power ...!

Resistance exercise seemed to be easier to tolerate, probably due to the break in intensity between sets. I still had to force myself to complete my routine for the day. Each subsequent set felt easier to complete than the previous one. The heaviness sensation remained; for some reason I was able to push through with less effort. As bizarre as it might seem, nonetheless, I had to force myself to complete my training sets. On the flipside, my high rep set that followed seemed to go more smoothly with less effort. It was easier, but still difficult to carry out due to the lengthier duration in tempo. The best description I can offer is now I can look back on it as a period of physiological contradiction.

Meanwhile, the OTC anti-nausea medicine had lost its effectiveness. In fact, it became useless. While I gave into the nausea "I yield", ran through my mind as I recalled reading "Ivanhoe" back in my high school days. I needed a stronger drug. My stomach ached; I wanted to vomit, but dry heaved, instead, a practice which became commonplace. I saw it as another weakness I had to accept. More of my self-proclaimed invincibility lay by the roadside. As the treatment advanced, I was abundantly reminded that I had vulnerabilities and frailties like most everybody else ... I was human, after all.

My oncologist proved to be undeniably right. I finally called his office to request his anti -nausea prescription. It took me until the Sunday, the end of week 10 in my treatment protocol, to begin to feel energetic and as normal as the treatment would allow. Unfortunately, these energy swings were going to start all over again after each and every chemo infusion day.

To compensate for energy differences, I reduced my increases in weight to smaller increments. Whereas I customarily made jumps in the five, 10, or 20 pound ranges, now, the increases were limited to two and one-half and five pounds. Progress was slower, but it was still progress. It more reasonably matched how I felt that day or week during my phase one chemo treatment.

My chronological age is self-evident. Those horrific days were the first time I felt what I believed to be an old man in his 70s; I felt my age and I never want to feel that way, again! It was nothing to brag about, except against all reasonableness, I did what I wanted to do those several days in spite of my fatigue. Having completed everything I'd planned was the only achievement worth mentioning. I would not give in to this chemo. Later, however, I would question how wise my choices were for the physical wreck I became.

By now, it should be abundantly clear that exercise has been an important part of my life for years and I'm unusually aware when matters go awry in my body. Health and longevity has been part of the reason; I like winning, beating the "competition". Further, this health awareness and competitive spirit helped me get through this toxic treatment that most men or women wouldn't have survived without serious side effects. Some may not have survived at all. What's more, I firmly believe I may not have made it through the treatment as well as I have had it not been for my extraordinary physical condition and competitive attitude. I wasn't satisfied with just surviving. I demanded of myself the complete return of my health. It meant a dedication to learning as much as I could about the disease, treatments, meds, and what I was to require of myself, physiologically and psychologically. I never gave up on myself and refused to allow anything to get in my way of recovery. This conviction effectively managed my existence during this ordeal. It wasn't pleasant, pretty, or without some permanent damage as you will soon attest.

Integrated Medicine Center
Shortly after my surgery, I was encouraged to visit MDA's Integrated Medicine Center to discuss the adequacy of my supplements and diet as a cancer preventative. I went in October during my phase one chemotherapy. I was in search of assurance/reinforcement/validation that my choices through the years were good ones.

Supplements and several foods were discussed. My daily intake of about 4K IUs of vitamin D was under review. A vitamin D test was taken to verify how much was in my blood; 37ng/dL was well within the range of 30-100ng/dL. I had read that for cancer prevention, my count should be closer to the 70ng/dl range. Although, my current dosage did not obtain MDA's approval, my argument was strong enough to elicit no change.

Next, my vitamin E supplement was discussed. The use of the E form alpha-tocopherol was discouraged. Studies found that it had little to no positive effect in cancer prevention. In fact, there was concern it may increase a patient's exposure to the disease. I immediately stopped taking this E form supplement.

Soy and trace soy ingredients were questioned. MDA had little concern as long as I avoided eating major soy products such as soy milk, tofu and soy plants.

Tap water vs. bottled was a good topic. MDA agreed with my approach noted in my *"Fit after 40"* book. They added that when I carry bottled tap water, it's better to drink it from a glass or stainless steel container.

Meats, they maintained, should be eaten in the following order: seafood not fried; free range, organic poultry; and grass fed beef. The closest I came to eating beef was grass fed buffalo meat which MDA approved. Eating beef once or twice a week, at most, was acceptable. It was better to exclude red meat altogether.

It appeared my regimen of supplements was well within MDA's guidelines for cancer prevention. Even though, I was required to make some change, MDA believed my choices were effective now and after treatment.

Visit number two to the Integrated Medicine Center was to discuss my diet. The dietician was impressed with how healthy I ate. Nonetheless, I needed to eat a larger array of colors in my plant-based portions. It was to ensure I was benefiting from the various phytonutrients by eating a variety of plants. I was praised for the different plant foods I ate each day: fruits, vegetables, nuts, and whole grains. I needed to limit my portions of fish, poultry, eggs, dairy products, and buffalo meat to about one-fourth my plate. I should aim for six to eight servings of vegetables and fruits each day. These recommendations are mentioned earlier in my book and I was delighted what I would recommend closely matched MDA's advice.

If we use the frying pan, we sautéed the foods in olive oil; there's no frying in other oils. With the exception of vegetable and mango juices, we strictly eat whole fruits and vegetables.

Although eating fish was a better choice than buffalo meat, I've had to be more aware of seafood high in omega-6 fatty acids. I was instructed omega-6 foods should be avoided.

For a sweetener, MDA suggested Stevia. I've used it since; it takes getting used to because its flavor is weaker than ordinary artificial sweeteners and sugar.

All in all, I had experienced an excellent sharing of information with MDA's Integrated Medicine Center doctor and dietician. I felt proud my choices earlier in life aligned so well with their cancer prevention philosophy. As a result, I've had to make fewer changes than ordinary had I not developed such decent nutritional habits so many years ago. Chalk another good choice up for Bovaird!

Chapter
VIII
Chemotherapy

Phase One Chemo

As you know, October 1st was the magic day when my wonderful experience with chemotherapy began. That first visit and every subsequent infusion, as was customary, blood pressure, rest heart rate, temperature, and body weight was taken.

My BP hovered around 141/ 82, a pressure I'd never seen in my life until now! The good news was it had dropped to my customary 127/ 65 range by the time my chemo rounds began. My heart wasn't working so hard anymore; it went from high range between 77-84bpm to a normal of 47-53bpm. Those change in numbers filled me with gratitude; I didn't want my heart to work any harder than was necessary.

This good news definitely had a positive effect on my outlook and well-being. I cannot imagine how I would have felt if it were the contrary. I insist that I was a very fortunate man. Yes, I put off being diagnosed, but commonsense kicked in and I was saved.

Each infusion day I was instructed to apply a topical anesthesia over the portal site about 40 minutes before injections began. A CBC blood test had to be drawn before each infusion to determine how well my body was tolerating the treatment. Time was purposely taken to ensure I was physically capable before that day's procedure. To begin, a saline solution was injected through the portal site to ensure the line leading to my heart was clear. Then, a steroid called Dexamethasone was administered to eliminate nausea. Finally, the chemical called Taxol, 80mg/m2 of it was infused each of the 12 treatment weeks. The entire procedure took about two hours.

Several nurses told me on my first day that the effect of the anti-nausea steroid would last up to two days. I should be aware of the change and prepared to take a prescribed anti-nausea medication when the effect wore off. My energy level the evening of my chemo day might cause me to stay up nearly all night. I was warned.

In fact, the first three infusion weeks, I was awake the majority of that first night. I made good use of my awake time by completing small projects at home.

Late October was the start of hair loss; I was losing it all over: head, nasal passages, body, and pubic. I began to look like a retired, impotent porn star as hairlessness became normal for me. My knees became especially bald, appearing extraordinarily different in their new look.

The oncology nurses' warning was right on; the steroid effect lasted no more than a couple of days. It certainly had a positive effect on my energy! I didn't feel like sleeping the first or second night. But when it wore off, I suffered a mild nauseous feeling enough to make me lose interest in food especially meats. It didn't matter what kind it was, I just could not put up with the scent or thought of eating it. So, I'd force feed to get some nutrition when my system tolerated it. As my treatment progressed, I decided it wiser to stop forcing myself into doing something my body was naturally rejecting.

There was a change in the odor of my urine as well. It got stronger which made me wonder whether I was passing off some of the chemo toxins rejected by my body. No one could tell me for certain.

As the month of October neared its end, I lost interest in sex. I questioned where it went and got the most nonchalant answer from my oncologist I'll always be remembered, "Sorry, can't do anything about that!" For a man who had been sexually active most of my life, the loss of my libido was catastrophic. I was concerned about my prostate and whether the accumulation of fluid would become carcinogenic in light of this change.

Little did I know my interest in sex was not to return for nearly eight months. What's more, it didn't help I had been off my testosterone injections, either. They were to resume in February, with permission from my oncologist, at a low dosage of 0.5cc every two weeks. I was fearful my low "T" would produce hormonal imbalance, again, which was the reason I got breast cancer in the first place. Age was another factor.

Chemo was going well for the first few doses until I began to notice nausea and fatigue with regularity. Along with these unpleasant side effects and for a guy with a fit core, my equilibrium seemed to waver like I've had too many drinks. I became self-conscious of a tendency to stagger. My footing seemed unsteady; I found myself having to be vigilant about my balance and stability. I wondered if there was no end to this wonderful experience called chemotherapy!

Just before my ninth juicing, I had my worst chemo experience. I hadn't yet taken MDA's prescribed anti-nausea medicine. Mind you, I stubbornly hung onto the notion my over the counter brand would suffice. It did until that week after I got the "double-whammy" message I needed something stronger!

I was nauseous and everything I did to combat the queasiness (Refer to Chapter VII) was useless. I was beat up and nobody had even swung at me. The feelings of what I thought a man of 73 would feel and behave like were uncharacteristic of me. I hoped this "old man' physical state of mind would be my first and last time facing it; I didn't like it one bit!

Phase One Side Effects

The frequent nausea and fatigue had not let up since they began. They drained me, took color from my face, and made me into a man who merely existed instead of living life. Under chemotherapy's influence, I was forced to see my personal frailties and limitations. This new reality humanized me in less than 12 weeks. No longer was I a man of indestructibility and strength. Would any reasonable part of this man ever return?

Often on my chemo-infusion days, I was asked whether I'd any falls. I laughed at the question until I realized I've had to maintain vigilance over my balance as treatment advanced. It seemed one side effect had been avoided thus far; a loss of equilibrium brought on by the chemotherapy. There had been times when I could potentially have taken a fall. Due to my core strength, and balance awareness, however, I'd prevented serious injury from falling. Until about a month after my phase two chemo treatment, I had to be conscious of my equilibrium to ensure it remained intact. What's more, I contribute the strength of my core and sense of equilibrium as a proactive/preventative step ensuring my balance and awareness continued as they had before treatment.

Sometime after my third infusion, I began to get mild nose bleeds with regularity. My nostrils would crust during the day and overnight. By morning when mucus loosened, so would the crusts of blood which were accompanied by light spotting of fresh blood. The whole ordeal was nasty! After several bouts of clearing my nasal passages, mucus would finally dissipate. The mild bleeding would continue throughout the day and night; I had to frequently clear my head of the dry-crusted blood. Interestingly, the matter never interfered with my breathing or sleep. I'd blow the dried gunk out when it was needed and continue on. My chemotherapist said my mucus membranes were affected by the Taxol infusions and recommended an OTC saline nasal spray. Although, the saline solution gave some relief, it took 51 days after my last Taxol injection on December 17th before the bleeding ultimately stopped.

My sense of smell became stronger; I would almost gag when the least bit of perfume or cologne filled the air. The aroma of food worsened my nausea. These bouts never reached the point of vomiting, but just enough to produce that nauseating feeling in my gut. I began to thoroughly understand a dog's amazing sense of smell. Some have an olfactory sense 50 times greater than humans. To compensate, one unique trait they have is the ability to cancel a scent by blowing it out in one concentrated, swift burst of air through their nose like that Boxer did when he was finished whiffing my chest in July, 2012. There were many times during my treatment I wished I could cancel a scent like a dog. I even tried the dog "cancelling" method, except it didn't work. Picking up scents got so bad I tried breathing through my mouth. When I eventually "tasted" the scent, I returned to breathing through my nose to avoid feeling sick to my stomach.

During this same time, I started losing a large amount of head and body hair. Shaving had become quite easy and less frequent. For about a week straight, I collected large clumps of hair from the drain screen after I showered. I refused to wear a hat and never considered shaving my head.

I was cautioned about tingling at the ends of my toes. I think it was infusion week seven when it happened. I felt several pulsating bouts of this sensation the day of my chemo as I settled down at night to sleep. Then, again, it interrupted an otherwise uneventful sleep during week thirteen. I had not experienced this sensation again since that time.

I cannot remember when it started, but I recall a phenomenon I had never encountered while working out until now. I suddenly realized I hardly perspired during my aerobic core and interval training workouts. It must have been the Taxol because two weeks after my last infusion, I began sweating, normally, again. Either I retained a lot of water or it was passed off.

Nevertheless, these bouts of not perspiring remain a mystery to this day, I recall drinking a lot of fluids especially tap water, back then, and, yet, did not profusely perspire during these types of workouts.

My energy level on bad days had nearly incapacitated me, altogether. I didn't feel like doing anything, but sit or sleep. My strength was reduced to about 40 per cent in the gym. My aerobic interval training was significantly impacted.

Two days before surgery. August 29, 2012, my rest speed was 5.1 mph while my work speed was between 6.7-7.3 mph. During the chemo days, I'd gone down to a blistering 3.7 mph and 4.9 mph, respectively. Chemotherapy beat the heck out of me! Even on my "good" days, my energy level might have hovered around 80%.

Calf strength had remained relatively constant. Most any calf exercise I did, I've very closely matched what I'd done before my surgery in 2012. Conversely, biceps and triceps were impacted the hardest; they're at about the 30-40% strength range.

About infusion week eleven, I noticed my finger nails felt very sensitive as though I'd cut them too short when I haven't cut them at all. If I pressed down on the top of them, they felt as if I jammed them in a door. Buttoning my shirts and tearing paper became a painful experience, but still part of everyday living.

A closer look revealed a bloody deposit of some kind accumulating in clusters beneath the central bottom part of my nails. There seemed to be hemorrhaging when none at all had started. The discoloration was more pronounced on my thumb, index and middle fingers than the remaining two on each hand.

My chemo-therapist explained this effect was brought on by the Taxol and it would be cumulative as the infusions progressed. This buildup of red-like substance was actually bloody pus that eventually stopped after my 12th week of treatment.

As my fingernails grew, the pus dried and moved towards the top of each nail. I'd, then, scrape as much of this bloody gunk from underneath as I could. My scraping left large gaps which caused my fingertips to feel sensitive all over, again, like I'd cut each nail too close to the skin line. My fingernails didn't feel normal, again, until August, 2013, almost a year later. In the meantime, I had to be careful handling anything I picked up to minimize the discomfort at my fingertips.

This puss-effect prompted me to check my toe nails. Sure enough, they had the same sensation, but were less sensitive to the touch. It might have been because they had a thicker nail. Where my fingernails kept their color, my toe nails appeared to take on a gray/purple tint. What's more, I saw no blood spotting or clustering as was common underneath my fingernails. Interestingly, my two big toes nails seemed to be the only ones affected.

With a PSA of 1.4 and a slightly enlarged prostate, my nightly trips to the rest room were minimal (zero to once a night) until chemotherapy. As I usually did, I drink a lot of water especially after my aerobic workouts. To get up from bed twice a night was considered exceptional. Now, four times a night with regularity was the norm which wreaked havoc with my uninterrupted sleep. Due to these interruptions, my time in bed had significantly increased.

Emptying my bladder became an issue; I had to consciously apply pressure to be assured of fully emptying at each bathroom visit. This practice became commonplace during treatment. Additionally, I noticed this frequency was likely to recur during the first week of each infusion. The passage of so much fluid, might explain how my body was ridding itself of the toxins from my workouts and a compensation for not perspiring when I was at the gym.

As a rule, I'd needed close to nine hours of quality sleep to completely recover from an intense workout before chemo. It had been my usual sleep duration since I began training. Now, I can get by sometimes with less than seven hours without feeling tired the next morning.

My post workout experience was different during this period. I didn't feel much of the lactic acid buildup I'd typically feel after a hard workout. My intensity level remained the same, yet, I experienced little to no muscle soreness the next day. At this point, I had not taken calcium lactate (typically utilized to chemically remove lactic acid buildup after a workout) since before surgery.

I believe it had everything to do with my treatment. Chemo was intended to restrict or retard any fast growing cell whether it was cancerous or healthy; it did not distinguish the tissues. I wondered whether fast growing cells included any rebuilding of muscle fibers following a workout. Dr. Kovitz, my oncologist, could not confirm such a claim since no documented studies included the retardation of muscle fiber cell rebuilding.

I'd also include fat cell retardation not documented in any of the studies. During my treatment, I was chemically very different. I'd junked out several times, yet, my waist got smaller, down to 32 from 33 inches. I didn't put on the fat, although, I'm not genuinely trying to add it on, either. Whether my core aerobic and treadmill routines had much to do with countering my junking out could not be answered.

Moreover, my appetite had been significantly affected by the nausea and could explain my slow weight gain. Chemo was administered on Monday mornings. As infusions progressed, I could plan on feeling nauseous by the following evening as the anti-nausea steroid wore off. Thus, I began my anti-nausea prescription on Monday and continued it until Friday. Although, it quieted my stomach, my appetite did not completely return until three to four days later following infusion. When I start feeling nauseous, my sense of smell went way up. Just looking at most foods including meat turned my stomach. I'd get very selective about what I ate and oft times tried to force feed when I believed it was better for my health. Unfortunately, I was unsuccessful with this notion and stopped trying to do something my body resisted. After all, there had to be a reason for my system rejecting food.

I read my MD Anderson 12-27-2012 Chemotherapist's Report online via mymdanderson.com. My chemotherapist, Dr. Craig Kovitz, reported that I'd handled the treatment quite well. *"This patient has continued and now completed Taxol chemotherapy, 12 weekly doses at 80 mg/m2. He has done extremely well without any acute issues except for the fact that he now notes some numbness* (it was tenderness) *at his fingertips, which has occurred over the past 1-2 weeks along with nail bed changes with pigment changes, which he has noticed as well* (If you pressed on the nails, it felt like they were jammed in a door.). *He otherwise has not had any acute complaints ... He is an extremely physically active man and has had to cut back some on his workouts. His performance status still remains a 0-1. He has reported no nausea, vomiting, diarrhea, chest pain, focal neurologic complaints, or other acute issues."*

My nose was, now, draining a lot during and after meals. Since there were no nasal hairs to catch the slow flow of mucus, it drained and drained. I had to make certain there was enough tissue on hand to clear my head before the fluid drizzled onto my face and possibly my food. I never realized until then one of the functions of nostril hairs. When they trap dripping mucus, it has time to solidify. These hardened masses, then, are cleared out by conventional nose blowing throughout the day. The absence of nasal hair could also explain why infants needed their nose wiped so often while they ate their meals in their high chair, no nasal hairs.

My remaining head hair, although, growing ever so slowly, appeared to be getting denser on top late in my phase one chemotherapy. Contrary to my chemotherapist's prediction, I did not lose all my hair. I did lose most of it on top where it has remained short. Haircuts became less expensive. I'd get a trim once every five to six weeks instead my standard two week intervals since new hair growth had been retarded by treatment.

Phase Two Chemo

The second phase of chemo got underway on the 31st of December, 2012. Timing is everything; it was a subdued New Year's Eve celebration, no alcohol, we stayed home and went to bed before midnight.

I had not been infused for two weeks. That treatment break allowed a glimpse of what it might be like to be off chemo altogether. Most of my energy and appetite had temporarily returned. However, I'd been told my internal system would return as close to normal as before chemo about four to six weeks after all therapy including radiation concluded.

Nonetheless, almost normal was how I felt at the time which was to say a significant difference from being on chemotherapy for 12 weeks. My workouts were almost normal compared to what I remembered from last August. For instance, I felt lactic acid build up afterward. I was perspiring, too. I could jog up to five mph without feeling winded, unheard of before this time and during phase one chemo. The weights I recorded to use in my routines got easier to handle with less fatigue in the aftermath.

For this wonderful round of new torture, three chemicals (**F** – Fluorouracil5, **A** - Adriamycin (the Orange Devil), and **C** - Cyclophosphamide) are administered every three weeks for a total of four separate injections. My last chemo day was planned for March 11, 2013. This infusion phase is nicknamed FAC for the three chemicals utilized. The Orange Devil described a discharge in the urine the first few times after infusion. It's supposed to be harmless and part of the dye from the chemical.

My first week's experience was not the most pleasant. Nausea hit Tuesday morning, bright and early and stayed with me for three days in spite of taking the anti-nausea medicine. Fatigue with barely an appetite became the norm, once again. I haven't had the drive or energy to workout. Not fun. By mid-day Friday, I thought, I was clear of anymore nausea. Still, fatigue lingered until Monday, one week after my tri-chemo juicing.

Lucky me, the nagging nausea returned, six and eight days after my infusion day (Sunday and Tuesday evenings), it snuck up without notice; thank God for anti-nausea pills.

I began to workout, again, one week after my first infusion. It was HIIT (High Intensity Interval Training) day on the treadmill with nine intervals to complete. After having not been running for 11 days, it went rather well. I perspired profusely for the first time since last year. What a great, aggravating annoyance to put up with once, again! The Taxol chemo must have a perspiration/water retention property in it as it has to so many other unpleasant qualities.

My first resistance workout followed the next day, Tuesday. I noticed my surgery arm range of motion was unsteady and limited after being away from weight bearing exercise for 11 days. That familiar perspiration accompanied this workout, too; I welcomed and embraced it like an old friend.

As the week progressed, my energy and strength seemed to return. By Thursday, I was eating quite normally. Speed and endurance were still lagging. My equilibrium slowly came back, though. I even jogged on the treadmill at five mph without fatigue as I'd been accustomed. I was breathing normally and my recovery time seemed shorter. With some caution in saying it aloud, I felt my endurance coming back.

I had shaven Wednesday evening and could begin to feel stubble by Friday, an unusual occurrence since last summer. This round of treatment might not be so bad after the first five or six days, I concluded.

The 12th day out was a relatively warm January Houston evening (72degrees F) and a bit humid as well. I'd just taken our dog out for the last time (about 10pm). As I re-entered our home, I began to perspire profusely; the first time since last summer. Although, I had to reacquaint myself with the discomfort, I greeted it with open arms. This feeling of getting back to normal was exhilarating; I just hoped there was no more cancer in me, then, I'd feel my very best.

My second infusion was handled more wisely. I took my anti-nausea medication the evening of the infusion. Plus, I began to take a ginger laced candy to minimize any remaining upset stomach. I hadn't felt as sickly nor has my energy been sapped as it had been after the first infusion. I still had my appetite, but I was cautious about how much and what I ate.

I took it easy on my first resistance workout. It happened to be the evening of the same day of my infusion. I planned to go up to 25 reps on my training set, nothing heavy just to see how I'd feel. What's this? I didn't feel drained or hammered? In fact, it went quite well; the entire week was surprisingly less eventful than the first...

Two days after my second infusion, however, I had one of the biggest scares of my life. As I was out on morning errands; my vision got extraordinarily blurred and cloudy while driving on the highway. The glare from the sun was fierce; I got scared, but remained in control. I couldn't read street signs, find stop signs, or make out automobile license numbers in front of me. I was helplessly in danger; I'd never encountered anything like this particular effect before. All errands were completed as planned, but it was a struggle to drive back home, safely.

Since it happened so quickly after the second juicing, my fiancé and I grew suspicious. It may have been caused by one of the three infusion chemicals. We surfed the Net to find Fluorouracil5, the **F** chemical in the FAC trifecta, was used. It appeared to be the culprit.. It Way down the list under Rare Side Effects was blurred vision. Now, what was I to do? How permanent was this?

As the days, passed, my vision improved ever so slightly. Too, I found that I could see much better on overcast days when the sun's glare was at a minimum. My UV filtered sunglasses were a big help as well, but it was still a scary challenge each time I drove short distances under this condition.

Why would I drive under these conditions and wouldn't commonsense tell me to wait until after treatment? Why didn't my oncologist caution me of this danger? I didn't know nor was I told of this risk by anyone at MDA which tells me not all is evident and I had to find out for myself which put me in extreme danger the day I innocently began doing my errands.
I was able to see well enough for general reading. If the font was too small on my computer, I'd have to increase its size to make out the characters. I had trouble with contrast when it was too light. Until late May, I had to bold sections of this manuscript as I was working on it to see the type better. While I was online checking mail or conducting research, I'd have to magnify pages for easier reading.

It took noticeably longer to readjust my eyesight when entering a building after having been in the sunlight for a while. The sun's glare was very difficult to cope. What other not so good experiences do I have to look forward to?

My vision improved while driving when opening a window to look out vs. peering through the glass. It might have been a light refraction issue. At best my distance vision is only good up to about 25 feet, way below normal. In time, it increased to about 60 feet. The sun's glare was overwhelmingly fierce, quite blinding. I had to exercise extreme caution when driving.

The cloudiness in my eyes appeared to be in the lens. Without an ophthalmologist to verify, it was difficult to say what was causing this phenomenon. Fortunately, the murkiness eventually wore off by mid-May.

There was a mild brownish tint in my right eye, easily seen with my left eye shut. It seemed to be concentrated in the upper rim of quadrants three and four.

In talking to my physio-therapist who was treating my edema in February, 2013, a number of her chemo-patients had complained about the FAC infusions affecting their vision. In all instances, their sight was restored weeks after their last infusion.

On top of all this, I began to notice how much more pronounced my purple-white large toenails had become. I examined them more closely; they looked like they were rising off the skin on their own accord. Was this another post-Taxol gift?

Some 17 days after my second infusion, my large toenail began to lift off my left large toe. I taped it to ensure the sensitive skin underneath was protected until the new nail took hold. Four days later, the same thing happened to my right large toenail. I taped it as I did the left one. This chemotherapy was becoming downright freaky!

My third infusion was delayed a week due to low a white blood count found in my CBC test. It had been 27 days since my last juicing and my eyesight had improved ever so slightly. On a good day, I could read some license plates on the car in front of me while waiting for the light to change.

With the four week break between infusions two and three, I experienced favorable differences:
- I had a nagging, chronic hamstring injury that seemed to be healing better
- Recovery time from my treadmill runs was shorter
- My energy level reached its highest level since before chemo was started last October
- After the third infusion, I felt my energy level drop significantly inside one hour after the infusion.

About an hour went by from the moment my post-infusion procedure was completed and I left the Nassau Bay facility to return home. The moment I stepped out of the car back at home, I felt the energy difference right away; fatigue began its work on me, again.

It seemed chemotherapy retarded recovery and healing of tissue, indeed! Let's be straight about it; it impeded most everything.

My final infusion was 20 days later rather than the usual three weeks. I met with my chemotherapist while he reviewed my CBC; it was a go. My white blood count was in the safety range for infusion, again.

Since I was there, he examined a skin irregularity on my back identified in physio-therapy and concluded that it was unrelated to my breast cancer (Yes, cancers can appear somewhere else on the body and be part of the major contributory cancer.). He sensed that it was non-cancerous, but, wanted an MD Anderson dermatologist to have the last word. My consultation appointment was scheduled for June 14th.

Dr. Kovitz was quite vocal about how well I'd handled both phases of the chemo treatment. He had remarked, "Amazingly well", the day of my last phase two infusion. What's more, he thought my physical condition coming into and during therapy significantly impacted how well I've endured its physical demands. I agree and hope I'd never have to experience this torment, again!

I pressed him at a later meeting to explain what he meant by "amazingly well". He remarked I'd not exhibited one acute side effect: fever, diarrhea, vomiting, aches, chest pain, focal neurologic complaints, or anything else that would require medical attention.

Interestingly, my vision issue did not seem to be of significance which seemed odd since it was a rare occurrence. There's so much I fail to understand about this cancer and side effects.

Following my last infusion, the familiar nausea and reduction in energy lasted seven days straight this time. To feel better, I napped most of the afternoons. I wondered out loud whether my additional "sick" time was brought on by having been infused one day sooner combined with the accumulation of the other FAC infusions. The closest answer I got was "probably so". My body's reaction was evident. Moving my last FAC infusion one day sooner nearly doubled the days I experienced this wonderful touch of heaven called nausea and fatigue.

Phase Two Side Effects

During every round of this second phase of infusions, I noticed a pressure on my prostate gland especially during my extraordinary nausea-fatigue days. Just as in phase one when emptying my bladder, I had to consciously exert to obtain a good flow, very unusual and uncomfortable. Also, there was an unusual odor to my urine. Urinations became more frequent, up to four times a night which significantly impacted the quality of my sleep.

What's more, my olfactory sensitivity increased much like I experienced in phase one. It makes me think I have a nose of a German Sheppard. I get nauseous when I pick up the scent of cooked meat and other ordinary scents of the day. I didn't want to eat anything. To make matter worse, the pleasant lotion scent my fiancé used after bathing made me want to puke (Don't tell her …).

Nine weeks after my last chemo infusion (March 11th) the normal odor of my urine returned. I noticed it about mid-May which suggested that at least some parts of my body were coming back as closely as they could to their pre-cancer treatment condition.

All these ill feelings were constant reminders my insides stayed chemically skewed until all the chemo toxins dissipated or metabolized or whatever they do before returning me back to normalcy, again, as much as was possible. I was told it would take me three to six weeks to feel like myself, again.

Then, there was the bloody pus in my finger nails left over from phase one's Taxol infusions. These same nails were growing and moving the, now, dried pus upwards toward the end of the nail. Although, the looks were unsightly, the tenderness was most aggravating. Again, I got the sensation I cut my nails too short when they were just trimmed. Where pus once occupied a portion of my nail bed, there were gaps as the nail grew and scraped clean. Buttoning shirts and tearing paper was getting easier as my nails grew longer.

Finally, in April, 2013, some four months after my last Taxol infusion, my two large toe nails lifted completely off. The tape used to keep them intact had to be replaced each time I showered. Finally, the nails came nearly completely off, just hanging on by a small piece of skin. I took the rest off and examined what was left. There was healthy nail tissue already growing underneath. I left them to grow back on their own. I noticed the new growth had thicker ridges and irregularities quite different than the original smooth surfaces.

My body and head hair began to grow back in March; there was more dense growth in May. 2013. The top of my head was now abundantly covered whereas it had been otherwise barren for months. Some color even returned. It felt good as a man in his 70s to get a decent haircut and then be handed the mirror to see at a full head of hair.

My prostate seemed to be acting normal nine weeks (about mid-May) after my last FAC infusion. I was feeling less pressure on my sphincter. By June, all seemed to be back to normal, except no libido; thanks, Tamoxifen!

I had high hopes of staying on my workout routine and beginning my week with doing intervals on the bike following my last FAC infusion. Not to be this time, the nausea and fatigue was just enough to discourage any kind of exercise. I miss the feeling of a high intensity workout, but first things, first; it was best to give myself the time to adequately recover from this final infusion.

I kept asking myself, after this treatment was all over: the chemo, radiation, and five years of taking a pill every day … then, what? Would I be left out to dry, fending for myself? It scared me; I don't want to ever be host to any sort of disease, again! Following up on my questions, I learned that MD Anderson does well with periodic checkups throughout the five years of pill taking and thereafter.

Lymphedema

Lymphedema is a medical term for the swelling in my case of the arm and hand on the side where underarm lymph nodes had been removed. Since there are, now, fewer lymph nodes, fluid drainage from the lymph vessels cannot flow completely out resulting in swelling. If the lymph system does not drain, properly, the arm is at risk for developing lymphedema.

I began to notice this change during weeks nine and 10 of phase one chemotherapy. I thought I would have been exempt since I had fewer lymph nodes removed than was typical; I was wrong.

The cause of the swelling was my system attempting to use the removed drainage vessels that no longer existed and had instead had become scar tissue; I've had to learn how to mechanically move the fluid away from that part of my body through physiotherapy. It was a matter of retraining my arm to use other lymph node paths for effective drainage.

Another cause for the lymphedema was my own fault. I had my blood pressure taken and blood drawn from my left arm before chemo treatment week 10 which was a major no-no. Over the next several days, my arm and hand slowly began to swell.

My lymphedema condition will now always be a chronic part of my life, another fringe benefit of breast cancer. I have, though, noticed a reduction overnight from wearing the compression sleeve during bedtime hours. If and when I remove the sleeve for daytime activities, swelling increases enough to remind me my left arm will never be the same, again.

Immediately following treatment to ensure I did not create blood clots or other damage due to my oversight, I went to the main MDA campus to be examined and for advice. No clotting was detected.

Chemo week 11, I was reminded to not wear anything tight on my left wrist. Now, I wear my watch on my right wrist. Blood work and vitals are checked using my right arm, only. Employing this practice in the 15 weeks following treatment has helped get the swelling down, significantly.

There's something else about chronic lymphedema. When I don't workout, swelling tends to flare up while on the days I train, the swelling is more likely to go down.

I was scheduled for physiotherapy, February, 2013, to learn the proper method to move fluid away from my left chest, arm, and hand. In the beginning of the lymphedema process, my arm had to be in a wrap up to 23 hours a day. When I hit the gym, I had to replace the wrap with a compression sleeve. There were prescribed daily exercises, skin massage, and I had to go to MDA physio-therapy three times a week to get my arm back to as close to normal as I could.

Meanwhile, my blurred vision caused by the FAC infusions, although improving, did little to help get me safely to the facility and back home. I had to use cab service on several occasions to ensure I didn't end up in an accident.

As time passed, my lymph-edema condition continued to improve and was determined "normal" on February 27th. Good. Now, I don't have to wear all this gear. Wrong, "invincible-man"! I was instructed to wear the compression sleeve for the rest of my days with few exceptions.

However, I started on my own to determine how closely I needed to follow this daily regimen. Several questions came up: What's the minimal time I must wear the daily compression sleeve or keep my arm wrapped? What was the long term effect on the skin with wearing the sleeve so frequently and long hours at a time? No one in physiotherapy seemed to have the answers. The closest to a response was the sleeve had to be worn or arm wrapped up to 23 hours a day. They really didn't know …

As it stands, today, 2019, I've found wearing the compression sleeve beginning in the evening or putting it on just before bedtime and removing it when I'm prepared to leave the house the next day adequately suits my arm. Additionally, mechanical messaging seems to work when I employ two instead of the three prescribed sessions a day. And if I didn't maintain this schedule, my left palm and/or middle finger where it meets the base of the left hand would ache, reminders I must massage and wear the sleeve. Mother Nature just will not allow me to get by without doing these tasks … proving, again, I "can't fool Mother Nature!" no matter how old I am!

Chapter
IX
Radiation
and
the
Rest

Radiation Phase

Getting partially fried was next on my schedule. The radiation process was similar to being bombarded with strong x-rays with pinpoint accuracy intended to strictly target cancerous cells. Radiation is designed to kill these cells, shrink tumors, plus it's utilized to prevent regrowth and the spread of new cells. What's more, this treatment is supposed to avoid contact with healthy, normal tissue due to its precision. All this information is according to MDAnderson's website.

But and there is a "but", like most mainstream treatments, radiation is imperfect. It did affect healthy cells … my heart, left lung and lung wall. These "late effects" will be discussed, later.

Also, I learned from my radiologist, Dr. Stauder, radiation destroys some of the "T immune:" cells considered cancer fighter/preventers. This issue will be discussed later in this chapter.

In the interim, you may be acquainted with several common myths about this form of treatment. For instance, radiation won't cause you to glow in the dark. Nor will you become radioactive or hazardous to anyone else while undergoing external/internal radiation therapy.

On the other hand, some side effects felt during radiation treatment are generally manageable. Skin will redden at the radiation site. It will feel dry and itchy similar to a sunburn after several treatments. There could be minor peeling dependent on skin sensitivity. Changes in taste and smell can occur; foods normally enjoyed won't taste the same during treatment. However, on the upside, your sense of taste and smell will return when therapy is completed.

Another common radiation side effect is fatigue which can continue for several months after treatment is over. The level of tiredness is dependent on your physical condition and age; I did not experience fatigue after my last fry-day which happened to be on a Friday. When you feel fatigued, rest is the only recourse, submit to its call. Expect downtime napping during this phase of your treatment.

Besides making time to rest, effectively apply the seven characteristics to extend your life (i.e., diet, supplementation, sleep, etc.,) explained earlier. Drink plenty of fluids especially tap water. When you do all this, your immune system will be naturally strengthened while your energy level will return to its normal performance level.

Bear in mind, every man undergoing radiation treatment is going to be unique; radiation therapy differs from patient to patient. Thus, discuss anything that appears extraordinary with your radiologist. He/she can offer solutions to minimize discomfort during this phase of your recovery.

My Personal Radiation Experience

I met with my assigned radiologist, Dr. Michael Stauder to discuss my case. Friendly guy, I liked him right away. He was originally from Chicago and spoke "northern" English which I appreciated, immediately. It's a type of well-spoken articulate English I was taught growing up in western NYS. Dr. Stauder and I not only started off well, we maintained an extraordinarily good connection throughout my treatment. I always looked forward to speaking with him.

Our first meeting, he discussed my case analysis which determined the most appropriate plan of action to take. Since I had a tumor greater than 1.5cm (1.9cm) and the cancer had spread to my lymph nodes (nine of them), I was scheduled for radiation every weekday for six weeks beginning in March, 2013.

As treatment progressed, my chest began to itch and itch beyond the usefulness of the OTC anti-itch topical I purchased. I didn't dare scratch the area very much for fear of bleeding; my sleep was interrupted by the constant itchiness. A prescribed topical hydrocortisone cream accompanied by a special dressing to cover the area was recommended. In a matter of a few applications, the itch had gone away.

Toward the end of my near two months of radiation, I noticed another side effect. My chest under treatment looked like it had been literally fried. The entire left side was a deep red-brownish color. As long as I continued applying a moisturizer and the prescribed anti-itch ointment, it seemed to be okay, except for the color. I had the deepest, tanned near burned chest I'd ever seen including times on the beach or poolside. I was happy to eventually see this effect go away after treatment ended.

Throughout my chemo treatment as well as my "fry" time, I had online access to MDA's physician reports. It was important for me to understand their evaluations. Dr. Stauder's MDAnderson report disclosed I was an alert and well-appearing gentleman in no apparent distress who appeared younger than his age. His remarks reinforced the wisdom of my choices earlier in life to remain fit and healthy.

One of the few pluses to radiation was it felt painless and each treatment didn't take very long. The staff technicians seemed well coordinated, appeared to know what they were doing and did it well. I planned 30 minutes for my daily treatment which took less than one minute of actual "fry" time. Everyone seemed focused on one goal … to complete the process while adequately protecting my left lung and heart from damage. The left side of my chest and underarm were road mapped with different colored markers that acted as radiation targets. It seemed I had two iso-center fields where the radiation was delivered.

Every Friday following the radiation treatment, I'd meet with Dr. Stauder to discuss how well my body had tolerated that week's treatment.

At the end of my second radiation week, I met with Dr. Stauder as scheduled. Except this time, in addition to learning how well this week went, I wanted to discuss the immune T-Cells' study completed at the University of Nebraska (UofN) by Dr. Bilek's researchers. Dr. Stauder as a matter-of-factly said radiation reduced the number of naïve immune T-Cells in my body. These immune T-Cells were identified in the UofN study as the body's cancer fighters and preventers. Further, resistance exercise was found to increase their presence in the blood stream. Thus, I was encouraged to continue my weight bearing intensity training. No need for encouragement; it had been and remains my lifestyle, one I intend to continue for my entire life.

As was predicted about my third or fourth week of radiation, I'd experience some fatigue. It actually occurred after my third week; unlike chemotherapy, it was a sleepy-tired kind of drowsy. It caused me to nap up to two hours after each treatment.

About midway through the fifth week, I began to feel a significant amount of itching in the radiated area of my chest defined as radiation burn typical for this treatment. I was told mine was less severe than most patients and given a topical cream to quiet down the itch. Further, I was cautioned this burn was cumulative and I should expect more as treatment progressed.

Not only did I experience serious itching on my chest, I also, got a dose of chapped lips. I'm uncertain how it was related to radiation, although, I noticed my chapped lips healed after my last treatment.

The anti-itch cream worked until the following weekend when the itching reached a new high. My sleep was significantly interrupted; I'd lay there trying very hard not to scratch and wait and wait until the itching subsided enough to fall back to sleep. It would never completely stop. I'd lay there waiting for more of the same throughout the night, over and over, again, as the itching relented. Sometimes I would yield and scratch while other times I'd wait and wait. Too, I learned that my scratching gave little to no relief. I bled a few times which didn't make matters better. I was concerned how this bleeding would affect my treatment, moving forward.

Something had to be done. I was speaking at a conference the next Friday and the sleeplessness interfered considerably with my powers of concentration and workouts.

Since I had to be at the conference early Friday morning, I met with Dr. Stauder the Wednesday before my radiation treatment. Although, my chest burn didn't look serious to him, he called in a prescription hydrocortiszone salve to reduce the itch and accelerate the healing. What a relief it gave almost right away!

Because it was important to be well prepared for my discussion at the conference, I didn't workout the rest of the week. As a result, my presentation went quite well based on feedback received. In fact, among the attendees, an FBI agent suggested in confidence that governmental agencies would be keenly interested in my presentation after I add an advanced segment to further data gathering. Nice!

Meanwhile, I completed the six weeks with "flying colors" or should I say "frying colors"? My chest looked well done with a dark brown almost black color on the left side. The itching finally dwindled to a few isolated instances without applying more of the prescription salve. I was told I'd have to tolerate the itching up to two weeks after my last radiation treatment. Instead, most of the annoying itch went away inside three days following my final "fry" day which happened to be on a Friday. Then, it became a matter of getting the areas where I had scratched thoroughly healed. Also, I needed to put on a moisturizer to help with my dry skin.

Tamoxifen

The beginning of my final week of radiation, my oncologist, Dr. Kovitz, wished to discuss my use of Tamoxifen, an anti-estrogen drug. I'd be expected to take it for the next five years. That meant every day until May, 2018. That's 20mg of a drug I know little about,1826 days, but who's counting? I became concerned about the side effects especially anything to do with my eyes and libido. Dr. Kovitz told me I might expect some mood changes, hot flashes, and, possibly, other inconsequential side effects. He never mentioned my loss of interest in sex and belly fat I might accumulate while taking this drug.

My first dose was taken the day after my last radiation treatment. During the first month, I experienced several bouts of hot flashes, but no mood swings or other side effects I'm aware of besides no interest in sex.

With little to complicate my schedule now that my speaking "season" was over, I made time to research Tamoxifen. Men can expect a lowered interest and willingness to have sex. Great, I'd been sexually active close to 60 years and, now, this? What a significant change in my life! On top of that, it was possible to have blurred vision and develop cataracts. Haven't I had enough eye problems with FAC?

When I picked up my first batch of Tamoxifen, I read the attached fact sheet which validated my research. I, immediately, contacted Dr. Kovitiz's office for consultation and left a voicemail since it was the weekend.

Dr. Kovitz called back saying he knew of no cases of libido and impotence issues among men although there was a risk with eyes.

Loss of libido was serious to me. I miss the physical closeness with my lady and an inactive prostate gland could expose me to more cancer. Fluid buildup might become carcinogenic, then, cancerous. Carcinogenic material is the last phase before cancer and I don't need to be fighting any more disease.

Another fear I had was my vision would be permanently damaged from either or both the FAC infusions and Tamoxifen. Whatever happened to the "less than one percent chance of permanent damage" claim I'd been told when I signed the consent forms to undergo treatment? No one's standing up, now!

Several months passed and I'd lost all interest in sex. It concerned me a good deal. I know my lady and I are aging; nevertheless, physical closeness has been important to both of us. Also, I wanted to avoid prostate cancer due to an inactive prostate gland. To compensate, I'd been forcing myself, solo, to ejaculate. It was not fun; I felt it was necessity to keep my gland active.

Prostate Gland
I arranged a December, 2012 examination by an MDAnderson urologist; prostate gland health was of paramount concern.

Herein was the news straight from my urologist, Dr. Wong. Tamoxifen interferes with hormonal balance; it could be permanent after I get off the drug. If I don't keep my prostate active, the concern was not prostate cancer, but, a reduction of penis length and girth due to scar tissue buildup. This scar tissue could eventually prevent a full erection, permanently which is of grave concern to me.

There were several alternatives such as the ED drugs like Viagra which I stated had shown to be ineffective for me in years past. To maintain my physical integrity, a penis pump was recommended for use. I was instructed to appreciate its use and utilize it for about four months. Dr. Wong, also, requested a Doppler scan be performed to ensure blood was reaching my penis in a manner conducive to obtain a full erection. Further, he intended to recommend a tri-mix drug injection to induce an erection. All this complication because of an estrogen blocking drug I'd been prescribed to take for 60 months.

Unfortunately, I failed to follow-up with Dr. Wong's recommendations. I tried the pump, unsuccessfully, and believed that due to my physical condition, I had the proper blood flow. Thus, I didn't have the Doppler performed; although, one was done later in 2013 which validated my claim my blood flow was more than adequate. I never returned for the tri-mix injection procedure.

Remember that vasectomy I got back in '73? An article about vasectomies on webMD.com in June, 2019 put my mind about prostate cancer further at ease. It seems the non-production of spermatozoa reduces the risk of acquiring prostate cancer. Thus, my choice those many years ago was a wise one regarding cancer. It's also wise to keep the prostate gland active to minimize penis scaring.

Eye Tests
I purposely arranged to have my eye examination the Monday after my last day of radiation treatment.

The preliminary prognosis was not good. My doctor was somewhat baffled since I went through a battery of tests. He thought he knew for certain I'd need my right eye treated for cataract which would partially correct my problem. Although, cataract surgery was planned for May, things changed as the days passed.

What perplexed my ophthalmologist was the root cause that affected my optic nerve. I was ordered blood tests and an MRI to confirm/rule out possibilities like eye or brain cancer. All blood tests came back negative.

Then, I was ordered a Doppler scan of my veins and arteries along my neck up to my head. My eye doctor wanted to ensure I didn't have an eye stroke due to plaque buildup. Based on my low resting heart rate, blood pressure, and serum cholesterol, I doubted any blockage could be found.

The testing technician remarked it was good to have someone healthy go through her test lab. Again, test results were negative. Good. In fact, I watched part of the test while the technician searched for plaque and saw none. You could 'drive a truck' through my veins with no trouble was the expression I heard. My veins were that clean..

Additional eye tests indicated my lens was partially clouded in the fourth quadrant of my right eye. The tint was faint, yet, dark enough to interfere with close reading. Moreover, my distance sight had become limited to some 150 feet on a good day provided sun glare was controlled. Since my optic nerve was already damaged, replacing my lens could traumatize the nerve, further. My ophthalmologist didn't want to risk any measures that could worsen my eye condition. Being very conservative, he favored the ultra-careful side of safety. Nonetheless, I was advised to get another opinion from a colleague on his staff. It was not a slam dunk kind of surgery to replace my lens due to the condition of my optic nerve.

Obviously, there was uncertainty whether replacing my lens would improve my vision. My doctors just didn't know with confidence if it would work.

Meanwhile, my oncologist asked how it was determined the fluorouracil-5 (one of the three FAC chemicals in my phase two chemo) had precipitated the damage. All tests performed were intended to identify/rule out other possible causes. If they were negative, it narrowed the field down to the fluorouracil. Two possible conclusions were left: the fluorouracil-5 or the combination of fluorouracil-5 and Tamoxifen had caused the impairment.

What was known for certain; my right eye lens and optic nerve had been permanently damaged. What happened to the less than 1% permanent damage?

One safe alternative was to upgrade my eye glass prescription to improve my distance vision for driving. What's more, the health of my left eye would, now, determine how well I could see until a more viable solution could be found for my right eye. It scared me; before all of my treatment, my right eye had been the stronger of the two eyes.

Before my visual loss, I was told over and over I had a 0.60 to 1% chance of permanent damage from the cancer treatment. Those numbers seemed to be pretty good odds until after my impairment. I kept asking myself "With such good odds, how could it have happened to me?"

Post-Treatment

Eighty days after my last radiation treatment, I met with my chemotherapist, Dr. Kovitz, for my first scheduled post treatment examination. A CBC was taken and indicated I'd recovered well. After reviewing the details, Kovitz remarked, once again, "Amazingly well". These very words were used near the end of my phase two chemo; I'd become suspicious hearing it, again, like this and challenged him.

"Just what has made you say, "Amazingly well"?" Kovitz articulated although I had side effects, I hadn't had acute or severe ones like vomiting, chest pain, diarrhea, or neuropathy issues. He believed it stemmed from my physical condition going into therapy and how I managed my condition during treatment.

I discussed the research I'd done during the course of my therapy to better understand how I'd gotten into this mess. Further, I explained disease management was an ongoing lifelong task for everyone. Where I fell short was hormonal balance and age. After I stopped steroid use in my 40s, my natural testosterone production registered below average for a healthy adult male. It went on for 23 years, unrestrained, until I began testosterone therapy in 2008. More than enough time passed to create the hormone imbalance in my late 60s. Age, then, became the second factor. Dr. Kovitz listened, intently. I closed by saying I believed I got breast cancer for those very reasons.

I was delighted to hear his reply. Although, there was no data, research, or statistics to prove or disprove what I'd contended, Dr. Kovitz believed as I did that age and hormonal imbalance after steroid use caused my breast cancer. My body stopped producing adequate testosterone to support my activity and health which led to a chronic, long term hormonal imbalance.

Chapter

x

What Effects?

General

Early in my phase one chemo treatment, I was frequently reminded by my oncologist, Dr. Kovitz, I had a less than 1% chance of having any permanent side effects. As treatment progressed, however, and I began to acquire side effects, I was no longer reminded of this low risk.

As the number of permanent side effects mounted, I silently became very angry. I was afraid to assert the obvious because I knew little about treatment toxins, my chances of surviving cancer and the treatment. What the hell happened to my 1% or less?

I'm bitter and, at the same time, grateful for beating this cancer. I was inspired by the "1%" statement. Later, however, I resented those words when my fate turned out to be the converse. I grew suspicious and questioned how much truth there was there to that claim! I'll never know; what I do know is the indescribable rage I feel every single day! Was my extraordinary physical condition to "blame"? The permanence of what I've acquired will never leave me! According to legal advice, I cannot do a thing to the pharmaceuticals for what they've done to me!. It's absolutely criminal!

In spite of what I was told, my side effects began with chemotherapy, some became permanent! With each new permanent effect, I would beat myself up asking the same question over and over: "What happened to that 1% or less chance?"

Late Effects

Then, finally, I'm introduced to a new permanent side effect that may not occur until years, later: "late Effects".

About two-thirds of cancer patients have at least one late effect from cancer treatment. A late effect is a side effect that could surface months or even years after cancer diagnosis and treatment. Due to related treatments like chemotherapy, radiotherapy, and surgery, endocrine system issues may develop. They occur because cancer survivors are living longer after treatment than in years past; there is earlier diagnosis, assessment, and proper follow-up care to make this scenario more common.

Resolving late effects like endocrine problems and sexual dysfunction is important to cancer survivors. They can benefit from awareness, basic assessment, education, and being offered alternative types of interventions says Sai-Ching "Jim" Yeung, M.D., Ph.D., Professor of General Internal Medicine in the Department of General Internal Medicine, Ambulatory

Treatment and Emergency Care at The University of Texas MD Anderson Cancer Center.

Cancer treatment can damage the endocrine system resulting in a variety of thyroid, adrenal gland, hypothalamic, and pituitary gland issues. "Some chemotherapy can cause hypothyroidism, but the evidence is not so clear compared to the impact of radiation," says Dr.Sai-Ching Yeung. In his lecture, "Endocrine Issues in Cancer Survivors, Part 1", Dr. Yeung describes common endocrine-related issues experienced by cancer survivors, therein he assesses a study that best illustrates the course of development of hypothyroidism after radiotherapy. He, also, addresses common long-term complications of radiotherapy, states how fungal and thyroid infections can play a role in adrenal insufficiency.

Long-term cancer survivors, especially those with childhood cancer, have a greater risk of diabetes and obesity. Dr. Sai-Ching Yeung says "There is no clear data to guide a clinical management of type 2 diabetes in cancer patients and obesity…diet and lifestyle changes are fundamental." In his lecture, "Endocrine Issues in Cancer Survivors, Part 2", Dr. Yeung reviews recent data and key studies that show how some pharmacotherapies and anti-insulin resistance medications for diabetes as well as pharmacotherapy and surgery for obesity may be beneficial for cancer patients.

Personally, the permanent side effects acquired from cancer treatment is an unpleasant and unrelenting reminder. I would not have been so upset had I not been told a number of times that I'd have a less than 1% chance of any permanent damage. In spite of these assurances, I've developed these everlasting effects:

- My large toe nails were replaced with a rougher/courser nail. Not a big deal, just ugly looking.
- My nose runs intermittently during and after most meals probably because fewer nostril hairs grew back after chemo to trap and solidify mucus
- Strong urine odor. I don't know whether it was from the Tamoxifen or treatment.
- I'm forced to be more vigilant of residual injuries acquired in sports years past:
    - Calcium build-up surrounding my big toes – Football
    - Left ankle ligaments – Football
    - Left adductor - Football
    - Right knee underneath the patella – Football
    - Right hamstring - Track

- - These healed injuries are manageable as long as I effectively foam roll and stretch before and after workouts
- Left pupil has been frozen wide open and very sensitive to light - Second phase chemo
- Right eye –lens (Since replaced) and nerve damage – Second phase chemo
- Nine underarm lymph nodes were removed producing lymphedema from the left chest, shoulder downward to the hand – A permanent reminder to never put things off!
  - Fluid buildup from my left shoulder to hand which creates a swelling, unnatural appearance
  - Must wear a compression sleeve and glove every day in the evening to morning for the rest of my life to minimize daytime swelling
  - Must perform fluid movement "exercises" 2-3 times a day to mechanically transfer fluid out of my arm for the rest of my life
- No libido – I've had no physical interest in sex since October, 2012 due to chemo treatment which was compounded in May, 2013 when hormone treatment with Tamoxifen was started
- A layer of belly fat has been added since I've been on Tamoxifen. It's been a challenge to get it off.
- Surgical effects
  - Missing left areola – No brown area or nipple
  - Large scar across my left chest to underarm
  - Underarm puncture scars where drainage tubes were temporarily placed
  - No more hair growth on the left side of the chest and underarm due to surgery and radiation
  - Nerve damage to left latissimus dorsi near the underarm due to surgery – No feeling
- Hypogonadism: My testicles are about half their original size
- Prematurely aged organs and features due to chemo-therapy.

To me, these effects are more than disturbing, although, I've had fewer of them than most due to my health and physical condition. My hope is you've paid attention to the many points I've described to avoid worsening your condition.

What Can Happen Long Term
Several unsettling facts reveal what cancer treatment facilities have known for some time. The long term effects of chemo toxins on the human body are

significant. Further, in light of my findings, it's deplorable that treatment facilities fail to completely disclose these ramifications to the patient when they're required to sign agreement forms prior to treatment. For instance, heart complications may occur in some breast cancer patients following chemotherapy and radiation leading to permanent heart damage. This fact is especially so when the cancer was on the left side of the chest.

Due to a lower percentage of male breast cancer patients, the following stories/excerpts talk about women only. I was unsuccessful in finding MBC related information.

The following true story illustrates what could follow conventional chemotherapy and radiation treatments. Refer to this link for the entire article: http://www.everydayhealth.com/cancer/heart-problems-may-arise-from-breast-cancer-treatment-4626.aspx.

April of 2013 marked more than ten years since Stephanie Cirilo battled Stage 2 breast cancer. Her treatment began in 2000 and consisted of eight rounds of chemotherapy followed by 33 rounds of radiation.

However, the unexpected happened in 2009, during one of her routine examinations. Oddly, her doctor ordered several tests for her heart. Test results revealed Stephanie needed emergency heart surgery to clear a severe blockage in her arteries and to have several stents put in to prevent an imminent heart attack. Ms. Cirilo sensed she was paying for the aggressive breast cancer treatments received years earlier.

Instead of taking her PCP's advice, Cirilo immediately contacted her Cleveland Clinic Taussig Cancer Institute oncologist who ordered additional tests to be taken at the Cleveland Clinic. They included a cardiac catheterization and she was to meet with a heart specialist at the hospital's Cardio-Oncology Center that specialized in heart diagnosis and treatment of cancer patients/survivors.

When Cirilo's clinic tests came back, they indicated heart muscle damage directly related to the chemo. What's more, had she had the stints put in, she feared she might not have been alive to tell her story.

Ms. Cirilo currently manages her heart disease through periodic check-ups with her doctors and taking appropriate meds as prescribed every day.

Dr. Thomas Budd, MD, Cirilo's oncologist at the Cleveland Clinic, says heart monitoring is routine for breast cancer treatment/management.

Frequently, heart changes can be difficult to detect when they're not assessed by the appropriate specialist. "It can happen slowly over time, the cardiac function deteriorates," he states. Dr. Budd adds that if a breast cancer patient has a history of other heart disease risk factors, such as high blood pressure, he or she is monitored more closely. "What we're trying to do is to avoid compromising heart function."

A study published in the 2011 Journal of Breast Cancer Research (the year before my chemo began) found that among 63,566 breast cancer patients, cardiovascular disease was the leading cause of death. Moreover, clinical research has found that radiation puts breast cancer patients at risk for developing serious heart problems (e.g., cardiac fibrosis, an abnormal thickening or scarring of the heart valves) later in life.

Another study published March, 2011in the New England Journal of Medicine found the risk for heart complications increased by 7% per interval of radiation level. Further, women and presumably men who received radiation to the left breast-chest side, closest to the heart, had a higher risk for heart issues.

Dr. Eric Harrison, MD, is the medical director for cardiac advanced imaging at IASIS Healthcare Inc., a privately-owned company that operates community-focused hospitals in high-growth urban and suburban markets. Several years ago, he formed a consortium of health centers throughout the country who partner together to improve cardio-oncology care and stepped-up awareness.

"We're people committed to trying to recognize early that a patient is having cardiotoxity from chemotherapy before there are changes in the heart function," says Dr. Harrison, practicing cardiologist in Tampa, Fla. "We don't want the patient who is getting chemotherapy for breast cancer to have a cardiotoxic reaction."

Harrison said if heart changes are detected while a patient is in breast cancer treatment, there's usually some measure of intervention. Doctors may temporarily take their patient off chemotherapy, reduce the dosage, or prescribe medications for congestive heart failure like angiotensin-converting-enzymes (ACE inhibitors) or beta-blockers.

"To recognize it early, we have certain things we can do such as imaging and blood tests to test for biomarkers," explains Harrison. Tests include a more advanced echocardiogram, a type of sonogram utilized as a standard test for heart disease diagnosis. "These tests measure changes in the heart's form as it squeezes, and will tell us if there's any area that is lagging which would be a subtle change. You can't measure a drop in 5 percent with a regular echocardiogram, and you can't just go into any echocardio lab, you have to go to one that's supervised by a cardio-oncologist that would understand these limits and accuracy that's required for these tests."

Detecting heart damage in a breast cancer patient can be a challenge since many symptoms of heart damage (shortness of breath during exertion, palpitations, coughing, and fatigue) are experienced by patients as a side effect of chemotherapy explained Harrison. "It's hard to sort it out if you can't look for those symptoms". Dr. Harrison hopes future breast cancer drugs won't put heart health at risk, although he's unaware of any currently in development. Meanwhile, doctors must understand the risks and treat even most subtle of changes.

Nieca Goldberg, MD is the clinical associate professor at the Department of Medicine, Leon H. Charney Division of Cardiology and director of the Joan H. Tisch Center from Women's Health at NYU Langone Medical Center. Dr. Goldberg believes former breast cancer patients often remain fixated on the illness for years, even after they've been through treatment and have recovered. Some breast cancer patients may forget they're also at risk for heart disease. What's more, heart disease is the leading killer among women.

""Because more women survive cancer they also have risk for heart disease the way women who haven't had breast cancer do,"" she said. Breast cancer patients/survivors should take time to advocate for themselves she goes on to say, and ensure their heart functions properly via periodic monitoring by appropriate doctors.

Dr. Goldberg believes while having a specific facility specializing in cardio-oncology is helpful, ultimately patients need to be certain a coordination of care among their doctors exists for their health benefit. "We have to remember that when we take care of a woman, whether she has breast cancer or heart disease, that we take care of the whole woman and the treatment in the context of all of her medical issues," she said (as of 4/19/2013).

Although, Dr. Goldberg is strictly talking about women, I would hope these beliefs/measures would apply to men.

Based on these stories/findings, oncologists have known for years that certain chemotherapy drugs and radiation treatments can significantly impact heart health. However, cardiologists less familiar with these drugs frequently fail to understand their implications. Now, just over a decade, cancer treatment centers have begun to pay closer attention to this serious problem stemming from various treatments especially since breast cancer survivorship is on the rise.

Thus, it seems cancer treatment centers have been aware of what these chemo/radiation toxins can do to cancer patients especially those fighting breast cancer. They've known since 2007 at the very least, which infers MDA knew in 2012 when I was undergoing their treatment plan. Nothing was said of the possible toxins or heart problems that could be acquired long term nor were other disclosures made before I signed agreement forms. Four such forms were eventually signed by me which gave MDA four opportunities to disclose any of these unpopular implications before I signed. Instead and in every instance, I was told nothing!

How is this act a forth-coming, appropriate, credible way to begin treatment? My answer is as long as no one knows, it's okay to not disclose. Pharmaceuticals will continue providing drugs while making billions. I'm beginning to fully understand why the standard for treatment is five years; patients typically do not survive much longer. What happened to the Hippocratic Oath?

My Personal Late Effect
Research leading into my experience with late effects some four years after treatment validated what I went through. It occurred, in spite, of the documented fact my heart and fitness levels were above average for a man of any age let alone in his 80s. My normal daily RHR (rest heart rate) was and is typically 53 bpm while BP is in the range of 127/67. I've recorded workout heart rates since 2007. There was no reason besides the chemo and radiation for this cardiac condition to develop in me.

Mind you, I had nearly six months of chemo ending mid-March, 2013 followed by nearly eight weeks of radiation ending May 17, 2013. It was about three years eight months, later, when it happened: sometime in late January, 2017.

Ever since my competitive Olympic weightlifting days, I've journaled workouts to track progress, log what I'd accomplished each workout session, and anticipate change to avoid getting stale. On my aerobic and leg days, I'd either treadmill or bike for intervals or a warm-up. As a general practice, I'd record heart rate via a heart-rate/wrist watch immediately after my run, one minute and three minutes later. Thus, I've had a history of what my heart rates were following leg warm-ups/intervals for a number of years to record the health of my heart.

I'd read on two separate occasions (one in Men's Health magazine) some years ago that you should record your heart rate right after a run and, then, one minute later at rest to determine the health of your heart. If your heart rate has not gone down more than two beats after 60 seconds of rest, you can expect a heart attack within the next two years. I got all the incentive I needed from those articles to begin recording my heart rates some 12 years ago. I added the three minute logging to be certain my heart rate continued to go down after a jog or hard run.

There have been few times I've forgotten to wear my watch. In those instances, I depended on the treadmill heart monitor at the gym. Sometime and beginning in late January, 2017 … strange … I saw a few readings that were extraordinarily high. High for me would be greater than 170 beats per minute; I was seeing 183-191. What? It must be the treadmill monitor I reasoned. I'd never recorded anything that high on my watch. So, I blamed the gym equipment and since it's nearly impossible to use the same treadmill every workout due to the "first come, first served" principle, I thought little about it. Besides, it happened intermittently which caused me to believe it was the equipment

Now, we're in early February and my watch seemed to be recording intermittent high numbers which I suspected were errors. After all, my rest heart rate had been consistently in the low to mid-50s for years. Nevertheless, I grew suspicious. Why would my watch read high these few times? Could it be something else?

This particular February Tuesday, I was getting my hair cut in the same strip mall where I shop for groceries. They had a blood pressure-heart rate monitor for public use. After my hairstylist finished, I went over to the grocery store to check my vitals. I'd grown very curious since I've had no outward signs of irregularity, loss of breath, or feeling faint/weak. That is, except at times, when I got off the treadmill. What the heck is going on?

Good, no one was using the monitor. What: 139/79 and a heart rate of 99? I panicked; my numbers were never this high not even on this monitor! I measured three more times; each subsequent time, my numbers went higher to a final 141/89 & 104 heart rate. What was happening? No symptoms, no signs of irregularity, yet this!

I immediately got an appointment that afternoon to see my PCP! He thought it was hypertension. Not me. I don't get that way!

Next, I directly set up an appointment to a cardiologist clinic I'd used during chemo for the next day. They wanted to monitor my activity for about a day; irregularities were found which prompted more EKGs. Their diagnosis was I acquired atrial-fibrillation and fluttering. Without feeling "out of breathe", faint or nausea, my heart was, intermittently, fibbing up to 200 bpm and fluttering up to 400bpm.

I asked how possible was this condition caused by chemotherapy or radiation? With no hesitation I heard, "Likely both"! The nurse practitioner explained they've seen patients in this condition many times before following their bout with chemotherapy and radiation Thanks, again, pharmaceuticals!). Based on their experience, my condition appeared to be the result of my cancer treatment. What's more, my acquired situation validated my findings. Why didn't MDA disclose this possibility before I was required to sign those four agreements?

Mind you, I had an absolutely healthy heart and body going into cancer treatment! In spite of my stellar condition, it still wasn't enough to overcome all this chemo/radiation toxicity. Something had to be done to thwart the use of these treatments! This was wrong especially when the treatment centers know what may be in store for breast cancer patients in their future and still insisted these toxic treatments were the only alternatives to treat cancer!

Questions immediately came to mind, "Late Effect?"; "What was the wording in the agreements I signed at MDA? What was the statute of limitations of these agreements? What could I, legally, do?"

As I silently replayed what I'd just been told, I was offered two alternatives: Correct this condition with meds for the rest of my life or get a permanent fix. I opted for the permanent fix called catheter ablation (sort of electronic jump start to my upper right chamber that was out of sync).

First, I had to more fully understand my condition. It was not a physical disorder, but an electrical one. My upper right heart chamber was electronically out of sync with my lower chambers creating the intermittent fibrillations and fluttering. The amazing part was I didn't feel any difference;

the only means was to check the treadmill heart monitor or my watch as I trained. However, by now, my "rest" heart rate ranged between the high 90s-120s, quite extraordinarily high for such a healthy cardiovascular system! My watch could not record the fibs or fluttering whereas the treadmill monitors picked up some of the activity, ranging in the 170-180 beats per minute (bpm) range. I got scared; I had no idea at what intensity I should be training, anaerobically or aerobically. Every workout, I'd check and record my heart rate to make certain it didn't exceed 143 beats per minute (220 minus my age) until after the ablation procedure was done.

Meanwhile at the clinic, they appeared to never have seen anyone in my physical condition at such an advanced age. Nothing was said, but I read their silence (I'd been trained and trained others in my profession to effectively read people.). In fact, my readings were validated when I was asked, "What do you do?" which gave me opportunity to describe my regimen. Without saying the contrary, they seemed uncertain about what advice they could offer to ensure my exercise safety. Fortunately, I used prudence in my workouts and recorded my heart rate during each exercise segment to remain on the safe side of caution.

When I first learned death was a possibility several weeks before my procedure, I focused on preparation including additional prayer and an update of my will. Further, during one Sunday morning brunch, I casually looked over to Jamie to say I was ready to "go" if it was to be my fate. What's more, I was all right with that possibility. She didn't say a word … Her silence could not erase the concern in the background of her eyes as she looked through me.

The day before the ablation, I spoke to my priest and did a good "confession" to be spiritually set for whatever might follow the procedure, death, included. I genuinely felt ready and quite good with my preparation.

My younger son and his wife were scheduled to arrive later that night while my other son was to meet us 6am at the hospital. He'd traveled nearly 300 miles during the morning darkness to meet us there. What a caring family!

Now, the anticipated day had come and we were at the hospital; the procedure was scheduled for 8am, but we were required to arrive two hours earlier. We met our medical team led by Nurse Jennifer and the anesthesiologist after I was assigned a recovery room sectioned off by curtains. I changed into the wonderfully modest hospital garb and was mildly sedated, intravenously. Since electrodes were to be inserted into the main artery of each groin area, I was painlessly prepped and waited with my family until I was carted off to the "procedure" room.

Some three hours later, I find myself back in recovery as I was greeted by my family and Nurse Jennifer's medical team. My first post-procedure task was to sit up without feeling nauseous or faint; I was too weak and couldn't do it.

In the meantime, my blood pressure plummeted to the low double digits (65/30 range). I hear, "Call the doctor ... NOW!" Seconds pass and my blood pressure has decreased even more as I hear, "Get the ICU cart, NOW!!" As people scurried about, I knew this was a time I had no control. My fate was in the hands of my Higher Power; two words came to mind, "Oh, well..."

I learned, later, that the doctor arrived and did whatever he did to bring my vitals up. My next task was to sit up and stand on the floor without assistance. Nope, too weak; I needed more recovery time What's more, the mix between whatever I'd been fed intravenously and anesthesia were not tolerated well by my system. Nurse Jennifer and her team played a significant role in bringing me back from the brink. They did an exceptionally outstanding job!

I was finally able to look about the recovery room to see Jamie and my younger son wipe tears from their eyes. Truly, it was a trying series of moments until my chemical balance was restored. More time passed before I was wheeled to my room to rest for the remainder of the day.

I was released early the next evening with the harrowing gift of this experience I will always remember.

Mind you, I had an extraordinarily healthy heart with an exceptional resting heart rate and this still happened to me! I wonder to this day what if my heart hadn't been so healthy? Would I have died shortly after the rapid heartbeat symptoms began? Think about that question and your physical condition should you choose mainstream chemo/radiation treatment. Ask your doctor about late effects before treatment gets started.

My late effect serves as a warning of possible long term risks associated with chemotherapy and radiation. There are other treatment alternatives less invasive, safer, healthier, and less expensive. Unfortunately, many are unrecognized protocols publically considered credible procedures. Why?

Could it be awareness besides the lack of large scale advertising? Is there a strong unspoken reason these inexpensive alternatives are kept from the public?. For example, I asked MDAnderson "What other alternatives did I have?" in 2012. They claimed there were none with no explanation, remember? Could it be the pharmaceuticals, again? Meanwhile, patients are dying from these mainstream treatment toxins. It's got to stop!

Chapter
XI
Recurrence

General

Can recurrence happen? Yes and it did with me when I was diagnosed in July, 2018.

First, though, you need to understand several facts according to science and mainstream treatment, today.

There are two times in the human life cycle when the immune system is weaker than normal. Can you name those times? It's infancy and those of us 60 and older.

Secondly, when you acquire cancer for the first time, typically, you're an adult with a weakened immune system usually brought on by poor lifestyle choices, stress/anxiety, lack of sleep, and so on. Dr. Mark Lewis, formerly an oncologist at MDA, states you're more likely to contract cancer from poor lifestyle choices than family history. Also, it's rare when genes are at fault.

Cancer begins with a highly weakened immune system. DNA stem cells are exposed and some develop into cancer stem cells. In turn, these cancer stem cells grow cancer donor cells that spread the disease throughout the body forming tumors. These tumors can be successfully treated. When none can be detected during treatment, the patient is considered "cured" (Which is, in many cases, a big mistake.). You see, the cancer stem cells stay, forever, according to mainstream science and cannot be treated. On the other hand, according to a number of cancer medical professionals on thetruthaboutcancer.com, cancer stem cells can be treated (More on that, later).

Now for My Story

It started in the fall of 2017 when I was asked whether I'd gotten the flu shot, yet. My answer was a resounding, "No, I don't need one. My immune system is functioning quite well and I won't have to get the shot!"

What I failed to take into account was my age; I was over 60 yrs. old and well in the range of having a weak immune system. That's right, nature age discriminated me; my immune system was weaker than normal!

Sure enough, the day after Christmas, I got the flu. It was accompanied by a low level temperature, a slight cough, and congestion. I planned to fight it, myself, untreated. After all, I've a robust immune system (not realizing it had been significantly weakened by the flu). I'll be all right and intended to tough it out!

Big mistake! The symptoms hung in there until mid-February and were replaced by a chronic cough. I didn't think the cough was a big deal and still didn't seek medical attention. Jamie told me, however, I should have been hospitalized by that time; I never went.

I stuck it out; the cough lasted until the 2018 Saturday of Memorial Day weekend. So far, we're looking at symptoms starting on December 26th of last year and, now, it's late May.

As it was on most weekends, I was sleeping a bit later than usual/ quite soundly, too, I might add, when I was interrupted by a shortness of breath episode, Hmm, there was no cough; good, it's gone! I didn't think one shortness of breath episode was any big deal until I was interrupted three more times out of a sound sleep. Each time the shortness of breath worsened! I was gasping for air and panicking at the same time. These incidents were the very first times since birth I had any breathing issues! What was going on?

Then, again, this shortness coincided with my difficulty on the gym treadmill beginning January, 2018. It got progressively worse as the months went by. I found I had to go slower to warm-up believing it was part of the flu I had to get over and it would pass. In fact, one particular treadmill warmup had me literally gasping for air like an out of condition sedentary man! This breathing matter was getting quite worry-some!

Meanwhile back to the Memorial Day weekend Saturday morning … my chronic cough seems to have been replaced by a more life-threatening matter, shortness of breath.

What do I do? It's the Memorial Day weekend and my doctor's office won't reopen until Tuesday, three days from now! I'm afraid to go to sleep for fear I won't wake up.

Another first … since November of 1993, I had an anxiety attack! Jamie got scared and didn't know what to do. I was determined NOT to sleep that Saturday night thinking I'd never wake up!. Instead, I spent the entire night researching "shortness of breath". I can't go on for two more sleepless nights. I have to do something! At the same time, I don't want to smother to death if I fall asleep!

I survived the night feeling quite tired. I hadn't been awake this long since the Marine Corps many years ago. About mid-Sunday morning, I called my PCP's office to leave a voice mail wondering whether I'd ever get a call back.

He called back! Did you hear me? He called back … even on a Sunday! This weekend was filling up with a number of firsts! I explained my predicament to Dr. Plam; he called in an inhaler prescription to my drug store. He saved my life! What an extraordinary, personal physician!

However, how can I quiet down this anxiety? Dr. Pham wanted to see me Tuesday. He noted I'd lost a lot of weight, over ten pounds! I'm now in the low 150s, highly unusual! Pham wanted me to wait out the anxiety which seems to have quieted down and focus on managing my shortness of breath,

Well, several inhaler prescriptions later, it's mid-June. I got over the shortness of breath! Except, I'm still experiencing intermittent anxiety attacks.

Let's see, December 26th until mid-June, that's nearly six full months of the flu combined with everything else. I did it, survived with flying colors! Wait until I tell my oncologist, Dr. Jasani, at my six month exam later in June. I was sure proud how well I'd done.

Now, I'm at MDA and bragging to Dr. Jasani who didn't seem impressed at all. He immediately turned around to his keyboard and monitor to schedule a scan for July third.

My older son, John, came from his Schertz home as a show of support, accompanied Jamie and me when we went for the scan which went smoothly.

Oh, oh, I'm getting anxious, again. Several days had gone by with no word from Dr. Jasani. Is that good news (No news is good news!)? On the other hand, what's taking so long?

I've waited long enough, it's the Monday of the next week; I called! Dr Jasani hesitated … several nodules were found. A biopsy was scheduled for the 17th. I'm in panic mode; not again, please, no more cancer!

I cannot remember when I saw my PCP, again. I'm getting too many anxious moments, near attacks, and some attacks. It's time for chemical intervention. I'm scaring the heck out of Jamie besides myself and my boys …

Pham prescribed an anti-anxiety medication. It worked beautifully! All was back to calm! Meanwhile, my rest heart rate had gone up 10 beats per minute, 61-63bpm. I didn't like that and I've lost more weight; my clothes don't fit me! This med, I don't like being on meds if I don't need them. Pham wants me to be on it for about 12 months which seemed too long, but he knows best!

After the biopsy, I get the news two days later. It's stage four contained in the left chest wall behind my lung. There was fluid found in my right lung which clearly explained why I was unable to run/warmup normally on the treadmill. Please, not more therapy! Anxiety went way up scaring my son, John. He's only known me to be firm and a 'rock" of steadfastness.

Aaaaa, oooh nooooo …not again! John nearly rear-ended the car in front of us as I panicked in his front seat, screaming denial on our way to my home from MDA!

July 27th, we were to meet with Dr. Jasani to discuss a plan of recovery. I'm to begin taking 150mg of Verzenio twice a day, indefinitely, and injections of faslodex once a month. These meds were to stop the spread of and prevent more cancer cells from forming. I swear I won't be a victim this time either and was determined to find other healing alternatives to beat this recurrence! Back to research!

I noticed I'd lost so much weight, we had to go to Goodwill to find shirts, jeans, and pants to fit me. I was somewhere in the 140s, the lightest since my senior year football season in high school. I was down to a medium skivvy T-shirt and a waist size under 32 inches (the smallest since my nationals' bodybuilding competition some 27 years ago). Anxiety and cancer will do that! I hoped I could get that lean weight back; I looked terrible!

Meanwhile, we all agreed I needed a break from being home, a change. So, I went back with John to be with family in hopes I'd calm down. Due to Jamie's responsibilities at the University, unfortunately, she was unable to go with us. I'd be back home the next Wednesday.

The visit worked; John brought me back home feeling more at ease. John's a terrific son, all the travel he did just to be with his dad and Jamie! I keep saying to him his "reward will be great"!

His younger brother, Marc, is worth mentioning … He's got a wonderful full time job with a lot of responsibility. Although, he could not afford the time off, he was just as supportive on the phone. We talked as often as time and his job responsibilities permitted. I call him the "Prophet", he's become so spiritual in word and deed!

They and their families are utterly reliable when it comes to their dad. God Bless them all; I'm a blessed man!

With prayer, the change in environment, being with my family, and the anti-anxiety med all effectively brought me to as close to peace as could be achieved!. Now, I had to buckle down and research. This disease was not going to spread or kill me!

In the subsequent months and the chest-abdomen-pelvic scans demonstrated I'd made significant strides to beat this recurrence. My latest scan showed I'd been able to reduce the remaining largest nodule from 10mm to 7mm. The combination of healing alternatives and prayer besides mainstream treatment have all worked together to help my immune system effectively fight this cancer!

How was It Done?
One of the sites I've selected for healing alternatives I'd been following since 2017. That interest shot up when I was diagnosed the summer of last year, thetruthaboutcancer.com oft times narrated by Ty Bollinger and his wife, Charlene. I purchased their extremely helpful *"Ultimate Cancer, Prevention, Healing, & Healthy Living* Program". I also obtained from this site Chris Wark's information. He cured himself of stage 3 colon cancer in 2004. After reading his inspiring story, I obtained his ten *SquareOne* modules' videos complete with transcripts from chrisbeatcancer.com. Wark's modules were significant in helping me develop an anti-cancer diet! Lastly, I found cancertutor.com which has provided helpful information and validated what I found on Bollinger's and Wark's sites. In fact, I've found all three sites corroborate what the others suggest to beat cancer.

I want to caution you on one significant factor. Mainstream medical sites do not purport what these sites encourage you to do to rid yourself of this dreaded disease, cancer. MDA medical professionals, for example, politely smile at me when I tell them of several healing alternatives I've chosen to fight cancer along with their mainstream treatment.

Let's move on to the next chapter to see just what these lifesaving alternatives are.

Chapter
XII
Alternatives

General

The alternative treatments I'll discuss will be effective for some patients while for others, they may have to search for other means to help fight their cancer. This is especially true for the natural alternatives. They haven't been scientifically tested by widely recognized bodies nor have the number of successes been largely publicized. Thus, it will take more personal effort to determine what will work well for you.

Nevertheless, these alternatives have been known to rid your body of cancer. Bear in mind, I'm not a doctor nor do I have a medical degree or certifications. You decide whether these alternatives will be of benefit to you. What's more, as Mr. Robert Wright, author/researcher/founder of the American Anti-cancer Institute (AACI) has said what has worked for many with cancer may or may not work for others. It makes these alternatives a challenge to determine which ones will effectively work for you.

Additionally, I've included what I've done to minimize MBC recurrence in me as well as risks associated with any disease let alone cancer.

To be clear; the pharmaceutical lobbyists/companies have a strong influence regarding what is recognized as effective cancer treatment. Their billions, invested and profited may be significantly impaired if lesser invasive, less costly alternatives are determined to work better. Much is a stake, thus, they may try very hard to discredit my sources.

My recommendation is for you to independently investigate these alternatives online to form your own opinion.

My Second Question

Remember I left you hanging in Chapter IV after my first question was left unanswered by the MDA medical team assigned to me? What an awkward moment! Nobody appeared interested in the root cause of my MBC. What I had difficulty understanding at that moment was MDA was affiliated with the University of Texas Cancer Research Center. Why, then, wouldn't anyone want to research how I got this disease in light of my physical condition? I was outside the norm for acquiring MBC: Not obese, not sedentary; not unhealthy in any way except for MBC; and I had a stellar lifestyle. What an unbelievable start for MDA! It appeared no one was up for the challenge! Which begs the question, again, why?

After the silence was broken following my first question, I listened as my assigned team (one surgeon, nurse, and radiologist) explained in general terms my MDA treatment plan: Surgery, two phases of chemotherapy followed by radiation. Then, I was to be on a prescribed drug called Tamoxifen for five years. Again, the room became quiet as the three turned away glancing at each other while awaiting my response.

I knew very little about cancer treatment; I was warned through the years to avoid chemotherapy and radiation treatments due to their toxicities. "What other alternatives besides chemotherapy and radiation do I have" (was my second question)? "There are none!", I was told.

I didn't want to hear what I just heard; my mind began racing … What was my fate, mortality, and what about other unknowns? Talk about unpreparedness … I feared for my life! I wanted time to research alternatives, but was afraid putting off treatment would reduce my chances of survival. I didn't know how much time I had or how aggressive my cancer was. I didn't know whether my questions turned MDA away and they'd nix treating me; I just plain didn't know what to do or say! Reluctantly and helplessly, I gave the "go ahead" to schedule surgery and the rest of the treatment. I wished I had someone to advise me; I couldn't think of one!

Meanwhile, I had time to think and question whether these MDA professionals:
- Genuinely didn't know of other alternatives or
- Were instructed to say there were no other alternatives or
- Were influenced so strongly by big pharma the answer given was tainted?

I'll never know … but you can learn from my experience.

Then in 2017, years after treatment while still on Tamoxifen, I came across a highly reputable online source called "The Truth About Cancer" (TTAC). I was encouraged which inspired me to intensify my research for the benefit of those who, like me, knew little to nothing about this dreaded disease. You'll make better choices than I did; awareness is key. However, there will be those who'll refuse to believe my sources no matter how well they're documented. What's more, I've learned much of what's been revealed has been withheld from cancer-diagnosed patients. Thus, discrediting me would certainly benefit the pharmaceuticals.

Few Known Facts

Resulting from the effects of my cancer treatment, taking Tamoxifen as well as the late effects I've experienced, I've been driven to understand as much about this disease as I can.

For instance, President Nixon enacted the National Cancer Act in 1971 whose placating premise was to wipe out cancer in a short period of time. After all, Americans were told a cure was "just around the corner"; that was a laugh!

Here we are nearly a half century later and medical science doesn't appear that much closer to a cure. There've been donations/contributions made through the years to fund this cure, yet, there's none. No one knows exactly where these billions of dollars have gone. It's time for accountability! A reliable means would be an unannounced audit! The American people need a substantiated method to establish this missing accountability!

On the matter of statistics, there's astounding information referenced in the 2004 December edition of the Journal of Clinical Oncology (http://healingpathwaysmedical.com/docs/chemotherapy-5-year-survival-stats.pdf). A table developed by healingpathwaysmedical.com from this Journal suggests about 97% of patients who've undergone chemotherapy do not survive inside five years. Although, the table sensationalizes the effects of chemotherapy, its message is clear. Chemo is dangerously toxic. When patients must sign agreements prior to treatment, the cancer facility needs to disclose side/late effects and this recurring statistic.

What's more, breast cancer survivorship after five years has been marked at a mere 1.4% according to this healingpathwaysmedical.com publication. Until studies are developed strictly for men, MBC analysis will continue to be skewed due to the larger number of women in these studies.

"Most cancer patients in this country die from chemotherapy... Chemotherapy doesn't eliminate breast, colon or lung cancers, a fact documented for over a decade. Yet doctors still use chemotherapy for these tumors... Women with breast cancer are likely to die faster with chemo than without it" according to Alan Levin, M.D. Chemotherapy negatively impacts the immune system often causing more harm than good.

Moreover, Dr. Ulrich Abel contacted 350 medical centers requesting all chemotherapy publications. Data was collected and evaluated with thousands of scientific articles published in medical journals. His study, published August 10, 1991 in The Lancet, alerted doctors and cancer patients of risks associated with chemotherapy. Dr. Abel found the overall success rate of chemotherapy was "appalling" in spite of doctors still using this cancer treatment, today. His research disclosed that women with breast cancer are likely to die faster with chemo than without it.

Two studies dated 1991 and 2004 are 21 and eight years, respectively, from the year I was diagnosed. They clearly disclosed what the cancer treatment community has known for many years; chemotherapy is ineffective. It's criminal to insist on rigidly standing by an ineffective treatment; patients are being killed. What happened to the Hippocratic Oath ("… I will neither give a deadly drug to anybody who asked for it or will I make a suggestion to this effect. …") and physician ethics? The evidence cannot be disputed! Yet, not one word was disclosed of chemotherapy's deadly statistic prior to me signing treatment agreements. It's been 48 years since the National Cancer Act was signed and there's still no "cure" in sight!

Robert Wright, author/researcher/founder of the American Anti-cancer Institute (AACI) has determined cancer cannot be cured with a pill as many depend on this hope. What causes cancer is how our immune system reacts to chemicals (food/drink/bodily topicals, atmospheric) and exposures to various environmental radiations. I would add one more cause of cancer and that is hormonal imbalance. Some say genes can cause cancer, except there's only about a 5% risk attributable to genes. Lifestyle and lifestyle choices that trigger hormonal imbalance as well as the chemicals/radiation we expose ourselves to are the real causes of cancer.

Mr. Wright goes on to say when the therapy plan is to rid the body of tumors, this focus falls short of genuinely getting all the cancer. Further, radiation does nothing to kill the cancer stem cells; in fact, they become enhanced by the treatment and remain in the body, afterwards. Thus, what appears to have "cured" cancer has done nothing to cure it at all.

What's more, when cancer is detected a second time, the usual remark is "Oh, it came back!" when, in fact, it never left the body to begin with. Further, the cancer will be more aggressive the second time around because the stem cells weren't effectively treated. Why? There's no approved treatment for cancer stem cells. In fact, their existence is enhanced by chemotherapy and radiation according to many sources including bostonbiomedical.com.

On the other hand, Dr. Bradford S. Weeks says cancer stem cells can be treated. The target should be cancer stem cells not0 cancer tumors. He explains why science needs to focus on developing an anti-inflammatory that will stop the recruitment of DNA stem cells from becoming cancer stem cells for three good reasons:

- Only cancer stem cells metastasize (Cancer tumor cells do not)
- Cancer stem cells are resistant to chemo and radiation (Recovery facilities are not targeting the real culprit.)
- If treatment facilities fail to concentrate on killing the cancer stem cells, the cancer will return for one major reason. These very same stem cells are responsible for re-creating the cancer.

For additional information on Dr. Weeks and cancer stem cells, access utube.com.

Everyone will have secondary effects once they've contracted cancer. It can potentially come back more aggressively after conventional treatment is over. Without effectively treating cancer stem cells, the patient must remain vigilant of lifestyle and making wise/healthy choices after cancer has occurred the first time. Once the worst is over, typically, the patient will go back to the lifestyle that got him in this fix to begin with.

According to Dr. Russel Blaylock MD, neurosurgeon, scientist, editor of Wellness Report, chemotherapy damages body stem cell DNA which can potentially become cancerous. This treatment merely kills cancer donor cells produced by cancer stem cells and has no effect on the stem cells.

Although, there are no formal treatment center methods to kill cancer stem cells, there are foods/nutritional sources that are supposed to minimize/kill cancer stem cells. For instance, drjockers.com touts the "Top 12 Cancer Stem Cell Killing Nutrients". Some of these nutritional sources I've included in my daily diet. Give his advice a chance; every bit helps.

An Educated Change

It scares me for having been on Tamoxifen from May, 2013 until July, 2018! It's an estrogen-blocker that creates a hormonal imbalance for anyone prescribed to take it. I was determined to find a solution to this unhealthy condition. My research found that over an extended timeframe this hormonal imbalance can kill you. I wished to avoid all major side effects leading to death.

I reasoned that to maintain hormonal balance, it would be wiser to reduce the prescribed dosage of 20mg daily to some lesser amount to permit a safer level of estrogen (<40 and ideally 21-30pgm) into my system vs. entirely blocking its absorption altogether. I eventually reduced my dosage to 5mg, 1/4th the prescribed amount with favorable results (37pgm) much to the chagrin of my oncologist. In fact, he was quite frustrated that I wasn't taking the prescribed dosage. I sensed, too, it didn't matter to him that zero estrogen over a long period of time could be lethal vs. my healthier solution to maintain hormonal balance. Moreover, he seemed surprised with my knowledge of the matter and unprepared to discuss our differences with his well-informed patient.

Here's another question ... since MDA is in partnership with the University of Texas Cancer Research Center, why didn't they come up with my solution on their own?

Alternative Methods

I've examined several alternatives to chemo and radiation treatment. There's a technique called **ablation therapy** which uses heat/cold to destroy (ablate) cancer tumors without more invasive surgery. Special probes are used to deliver ablative treatments directly to the tumor. Computer imaging is utilized to correctly position these probes and monitor treatment progress. For details regarding the advantages, types of ablation therapy (i.e., cryoablation) refer to the MDA website. My objection to this method is it only targets the tumor and does nothing to kill the cancer stem cells.

Immunotherapy uses the body's natural defenses to fight cancer. White blood cells (T cells) that make up the immune system are stimulated in several ways by specifically designed drugs that cause these T cells to identify and kill cancer cells.

However, recent research has discovered several T-immune cell proteins that prevent them from effectively attacking cancer. MDA had found inhibitors of these proteins to allow the T cells to do their work. This treatment sounded quite good if it killed cancer stem cells.

Adoptive cell therapy (ACT) works in two ways: It takes a patient's immune cells and multiplies them into billions in the lab. They're returned back into the patient to more effectively recognize and attack cancer. The other method genetically engineers a patient's immune cells in the lab to recognize and attack their specific cancer, expands their number of immune cells and reinfuses them into the patient. These methods are undergoing clinical trials for solid tumors and blood cancers. Again, I say, for this technique to be successful, it must, also, target cancer stem cells.

There are other immunotherapies that fall into two general categories: **Targeted immunotherapies** and **Monoclonal antibodies** referenced below.

Cancer vaccines designed to help the body recognize cancer cells and stimulate the immune system to kill them are another alternative.

More specific to breast cancer are two therapies: **Hormone Therapy** and **Targeted Therapy.** Hormone therapy can help prevent estrogen and estradiol from stimulating the growth of breast cancer via oral or intravenously administered drugs Tamoxifen® is an example of a hormone therapy drug believed to be unhealthy due to its carcinogenic properties. Targeted therapies are drug treatments that boost the body's immune system to fight cancer. Herceptin® is a therapy which targets cells that produce too much HER2 protein present in some breast cancer patients.

The material, above is from mdanderson.org: https://www.mdanderson.org/treatment-options.html .

Remember, I asked about other alternatives in 2012? It's now year 2019; I've no idea whether these options were available when I was diagnosed. I'd, also, like to determine the success rate, survivorship, and chance of recurrence using the alternatives offered above.

To make better use of your time, I'll offer websites for treatment alternatives for chemo and radiation. Just how credible are they? You make that determination:

- Proton treatment: https://www.texascenterforprotontherapy.com/proton-therapy/proton-beam-radiation-therapy?gclid=EAIaIQobChMIhZysyPjy1QIVEHh-Ch1fNACXEAAYAyAAEgK5wPD_BwE
- This site offers treatment w/o chemo or radiation: https://hope4cancer.com/welcome/alternative-cancer-treatment/?gclid=CJjDrPX48tUCFcW6wAod_G4CiA

In less specific terms, below are several other breast cancer treatment alternatives you can check out. Cut & paste each alternative utilizing your selected search engine:

- IPT, Insulin Potentiation therapy.
- High dose, intravenous Vitamin C.
- Hyperthermia combined with radiation.
- Oxidative therapies.
- Immune system strengthening diet.
- Lymphatic Drainage Therapy.
- Chelation Therapy.

Lastly, an Australian berry called **EBC-46** is under scrutiny as a possible cancer tumor killer in humans. It's been successfully tested on mice, dogs, cats, and horses by cutting of the blood supply to kill tumor cells and boosting the immune system. Dr. Glen Boyle, heads the study as told to Australia ABC News at the time: Refer to http://www.abc.net.au/news/2014-10-07/queensland-scientists-discover-cancer-fighting-berry/5796106 and for a Snopes analysis: http://www.snopes.com/scientists-find-australian-berry-can-cure-cancer-48-hours/ .

Meanwhile, human trials have begun in Australia, http://www.anonews.co/berry-cancer-cure/ . Seek the latest news to determine the success and progress with human trials. Then, provided such compound is marketed world-wide, determine the cost and where it can be purchased, likely online.

However, I caution you on one very important point ... I agree with Mr. Robert Wright's analysis. When the goal is to just rid the human body of cancer tumors, the treatment falls short of completely ridding the patient's system of the disease. There must be a method found to treat cancer stem cells.

Natural Alternatives
For those of you who're curious about natural therapies, I recommend Dr. Josh Axe's website: https://draxe.com/10-natural-cancer-treatments-hidden-cures/ He explains 10 therapies he offers as cancer fighting solutions. Much of his site information I'd implemented long before I knew these practices were formally offered online. So far, they appear to have spared me from recurrence until July of 2018. I'll explain, later.

There are several other alternatives I've heard good things about. Although, I haven't tried the frankincense oil, I have successfully used the combination turmeric and curcumin. I put one tablespoon mixed in my anti-cancer salad which lasts about a week.

Proper dosage seems to be the big question and which application (topical, injection or ingested) is best. It's easy to over-dose without realizing it until you get sick. See what webmd.com has to say about the use of such alternatives.

Several books, outlined below, are for those who enjoy reading. What they offer may help someone you know who's contemplating cancer treatment alternatives. Bear in mind, the descriptions are from the authors' books. Titles are not included, Search online for them.

- Dr. Joseph Mercola: Advantages of the Ketogenic diet and how it may it help heal cancer.
- Dr. Rashid Buttar: How heavy metals in the body can cause cancer and what you can do to remove them from your body.
- Dr. Patrick Quillin: How you may be able to prevent and even heal cancer using the right foods and supplements.
- Ocean Robbins: The importance of GMO labeling, clean antibiotic-free meats, and reversing health ailments instead of fueling them by eating "clean" foods plus many more…

Foods to Boost Your Immune System

Go online to check out "Medicinal Mushrooms". You'll find there are more than 10,000 varieties of mushrooms in North America, alone. Some of them fall into the therapeutic category of medicinal fungi offering a diverse array of health benefits:

Turkey tail (Trametes versicolor) mushrooms are powerful antioxidant enhancers to the immune system and they lower cholesterol levels.

Reishi (Ganoderma lucidum) mushrooms help ward off viruses while facilitating balance in the adrenal glands and they promote feelings of calmness.

Shitake (Lentinula edodes) mushrooms possess anti-tumoral and antiviral properties. Shiitake mushrooms are so medicinal that herbalist Christopher Hobbs, editorial advisor for *Herbs for Health*, says they're effective for nearly every ailment: including immune disorders, allergies, candida, the common cold, influenza, and cancer.

Maitake (Grifola frondosa) mushrooms have shown in scientific studies to fight cancer and inhibit tumor growth. Additionally, they help lower blood pressure while balancing cholesterol levels.

Lion's Mane (Hericium erinaceus) Mushrooms are considered by world-renowned fungi expert Paul Stamets to be most beneficial in the world for brain, nervous system, immune system, and heart health. They also are known to improve cognitive function and help promote neural growth

There're also exotic super fruits besides these mushrooms:

The *Acerola cherry (Malpighia emarginata) and Indian gooseberry (Emblica officinalis)* have the highest levels of natural vitamin C, a healing agent for the body. Acerola cherry is a powerful antioxidant fruit rich in flavonoids like quercetin that support cardiovascular, immune, and respiratory health. This potent DNA protector minimizes oxidative damage and prevents the type of harmful mutations that lead to cancer growth and proliferation.

Indian gooseberries are rich in anthocyanin antioxidants that help combat early aging while stamping out disease-causing inflammation. These characteristics are combined with their rich density of brain-boosting omega-3 fatty acids.

Other foods you might wish to include in your anti-cancer diet:

Sprouted Seeds- Sprouting unlocks a cornucopia of seed nutrition that would otherwise not be accessible by the body. Seed germination not only makes seeds more nutritionally bioavailable while boosting their overall nutrient content.

Sprouting is especially important because it deactivates certain "anti-nutrients" in seeds that can inhibit nutrient absorption and even rob your body of its own nutrient stores. Such anti-nutrients include phytic acid, enzyme inhibitors, lectins, saponins, and polyphenols.

Fermented Herbs **are an underrated dietary element.** Examples include ***holy basil* and *lemon balm.*** Fermenting helps to break down and convert one type of nutrient into another, making it more digestible and palatable than it otherwise would be in its unfermented form.

Ashwagandha is one type of adaptogenic herb that's better fermented than unfermented. This herb provides medicinal support for the thyroid gland, adrenal glands, immune system, brain, and blood. Ashwagandha is an excellent herb to start including in your diet.

Tumeric and *rhodiola* are among the most powerful anti-inflammatory herbs in the world and their beneficial effects are greatly amplified when they are fermented.

The only objection I have regarding herbs is what's an adequate/safe dosage and frequency (/daily; more than once a day; weekly?). Moreover, how available are they, where and at what cost?

Probiotics and enzymes are supposed to be good for the immune system, except I haven't spent time researching their effectiveness. I mention them simply to offer you more alternatives.

Cancer Alternative Medicine/Sources

Dr. Manuela Boyle, Ayurveda mind-body systemic methodologist and breast Cancer specialist, has developed a natural compound from the coriolus versicolor mushroom to reduce drug resistance in conventional chemotherapies for several cancers including breast cancer. Clinical trials continue. It's known as PSK, a semi-purified polysaccharide used extensively in clinical cancer treatment. Several human clinical research studies strongly suggest PSK inhibits cancer progression and improves human postoperative survival due to a combination of immune system stimulation and inhibition of immune-suppressive cytokines.

Veronique Desaulniers, a breast cancer conqueror and physician/lecturer, says there're many factors to contracting cancer: Stress, depths of the soul; and healing of the whole body. She believes we have a lot of control over cancer prevention through detoxification/herbal use. Further, she says there are seven essentials in this process: food; specific detox; energy hormonal balance, exercise; healing emotional wounds/managing stress better; and biological dentistry. Boosting the immune system and practicing true prevention. Ms. Desaulniers believes when we accomplish all her recommendations, there's no reason to fear cancer

Tara Mann of Cancer Crackdown fame says there are natural therapies to rid yourself of cancer. For details, go to cancercrackdown.org.

.Jordan S. Rubin, founder of Garden of Life, offers natural, nutritional diets to ward off cancer. He's cured himself of cancer; read how he did it.

Dr. Axe's Essential Oils guide on https://draxe.com/essential-oils-guide/. There's also credible information regarding do's and don'ts of essential oils on webmd.com. I've read a little about them that mildly validates what Dr. Eric Zielinski says about essential oils in his book, "*Best Essential Oils for Cancer Patients*": http://drericz.com/essential-oils-for-cancer/. Frankincense, myrrh, turmeric, lavender, sandleweed, orange oil, lemon, and peppermint are examples in his book. They can be injected, ingested, sprayed, or rubbed, topically. Just how much is enough to avoid over/under dosing?

Paul Barattiero of *The Importance of Hydrogen and Water* says when the human body is properly water hydrated, the body will function more efficiently. Water is in every part of the human body: joints, brain, blood, and bones. In fact, 3/4th of the body is water when properly hydrated. When health issues rise, metabolic rate slows down, human functions are reduced, the removal of toxins is reduced, and the body becomes easily taxed/burdened. Read more about water in Barattiero's book.

Look for Dr. Stan Burzynski for cancer treatment innovations. He's located in Texas and has cured patients with tailored potions.

Liana Wern- *"How I Cured Myself of Cancer by Creating the Earth Diet"*, *"Alkalizing my Body"* where Ms. Wern purports five daily eating habits to heal your body.

Finally, check out Ocean Robbins: *"Food as Medicine to Beat Cancer"* – The New Food Revolution.

I recognize much of what I've recommended requires reading and you must decide how much research you wish to devote before a choice of treatment is made. My hope is I've saved some precious time before you devise a plan to beat this disease.

What I've Done to Prevent Recurrence
I'm going to begin by repeating the seven controllable disease management characteristics explained in Chapter IV that I live by to this day. In fact, unknowingly, I've practiced the majority of them most of my adult life, except for hormonal balance until I acquired breast cancer. Crystalize these contributing factors. How effective you follow them will determine whether you'll remain healthy or take an unhealthy turn. Online readings validate my choice to follow these seven characteristics to minimize disease recurrence (Refer to aarp.org; webmd.com, two of many sources).

What I've learned about disease can help provided you're willing to change parts of your lifestyle. First, as we age, our immune system is weakened by the ravages of time as well as lifestyle choices made through the years. I suspect one reason cancer returns is the patient's unwillingness to make permanent change to strengthen their faltering immune system. Typically, after diagnosis and treatment patients go back to the familiar habits that often got them into this disease predicament to begin with. There's always the belief "You only live once, so why not live it the way you want?" True, except if it's shortening your life … well, that's a choice you have to make. For every choice there's a consequence, good and otherwise.

Every one of these seven characteristics will significantly impact your life. When you follow a healthier lifestyle, you're more likely to have a positive outcome. You choose the converse? Well, life's certainly full of choices. I don't ever want to go through any mainstream treatment procedure, again. Do you?

Below is the protocol I've used to bolster my immune system and avoid cancer recurrence or contract any disease for that matter:

- Diet
- Supplementation
- Adequate, uninterrupted, quality sleep
- Effectively manage anxiety and stress
- Exercise
- Hormonal balance
- Lifestyle

All seven of these characteristics can be managed without drugs dependent on your willingness and discipline. I've done it for years to successfully achieve national ranking in three iron sports and, afterwards, maintain my health into my advanced age. What's more, your liver won't have to work as hard to keep you healthy when you rely on the power of yourself over prescribed drugs.

But, I want to caution you, life is imperfect and in spite of your good choices, illness can still happen. What I've described will minimize those chances.

My Anti-Cancer Diet
Here's what I eat to stave off cancer. Much research has gone into this diet composition from various sources: Chris Ward's SquareOne modules, thetruthaboutcancer.com, cancertutor.com, and several other relevant sites.

The bottom line? Eat non-GMO, unprocessed whole foods for healthy results. They comprise of antioxidants, phytonutrients while these same foods regulate abnormal growth and simulate apoptosis (the programming of cancer cell death). Plant food, fruits, vegetables (especially clean & raw), grains, legumes all protect the human body from disease.

Now for my diet ... I cannot remember when I've ever skipped eating a hearty, healthy breakfast. Typically, I have black coffee sweetened with Stevia (An MDA recommendation) with a deliciously healthy oatmeal recipe I've devised with nuts, muesli, crasins, blueberries, and cinnamon. Add lactose free skimmed milk to top it off. I may also have a banana (sometimes w/crunch peanut butter) followed by my morning supplements which are more effectively absorbed after eating.

Make certain your lunch/dinner meal portions are three-fourths multi-colored veggies/fruit and one-quarter your meats in order of preference: legless (Fish, seafood); two legged (Fowl, turkey, pheasant, etc.); and four legged: buffalo, squirrel, rabbit, and lamb. Beef is my last choice. I refrain from eating processed meats/cheeses. If I eat them at all, it's on my junk day with moderation.

Then, there's this "salad", unlike any typical salad comprised of known cancer preventers/fighters and eat it during most lunches and dinners throughout the week. What I put in this salad may vary, but I do not deviate:

- Spices: 1 heaping tbsp turmeric*; 1 level tbsp cayenne: ground black pepper*
- Crushed garlic: about 2 heaping tbsps
- Bunch of watercress/parsley as they come from Produce
- Sliced beets
- Shredded carrots
- Broccoli flowerets
- Broccoli sprouts*
- Diced celery
- Green/red*/white* onions
- A variety of mushrooms sautéed in virgin olive oil: Shitake; white button; and Portabella
- Hummus

I mix these ingredients together and serve without salad dressing, although, I'm told lemon juice and vinegar works well. I may vary by omitting some of the veggies for flavor. I eat this salad with every meal during the weekdays and vary on the weekend.

Be certain you access drjockers.com website to obtain what he believes to be cancer stem cell killers "Top 12 Cancer Stem Cell Killing Nutrients". Where you find an asterisk by the foods I eat is where these nutrients can be found that kill cancer stem cells according to Dr. Jockers

Also, these beverages/foods that I eat are included as stem cell killer foods according the Jockers: Apples, dark skinned grapes, green tea, blueberries, cherries, red raspberries, and watermelon. I eat these foods fairly regularly.

The following foods are likewise cancer stem cell killers per the doctor above which I eat less often, but do eat: red beans, eggplant, and pears. . .

Tap water (Filtered when I can get It.) is my main beverage followed by black coffee, green tea, and a variety of full bodied red wines. If I cannot find Stevia when we dine out, I've started to go without which reminds me to remember to bring some Stevia with me. Reminder: webMD says green tea is a good antioxidant source to lower the risks of contracting several types of cancers including breast.

I snack on healthy foods, only: fruit, deluxe mixed nuts, dark chocolate covered almonds, plain 70% or higher dark chocolate, low carb fruit flavored yogurt which I mix fresh fruit with to name a few. I eat with purpose which means avoiding junk foods and drink on my non-junk days and with moderation on my junk food day usually Sunday. However, I'm finding I only have about 2-3 junk days a month. It keeps me lean and avoids any belly fat build up.

I use the junk day as a craving reliever and to reward myself for doing so well during the week. I'm finding I'm having fewer cravings like I used to earlier in life. Moreover, I don't go crazy when I do junk out, anymore. Now, it's pig out with reasonableness of most anything I've denied myself of during the week, drink included, usually wine.

Here's a list of other beneficial diet sources you may find helpful:
- Dr. Patrick Quillin: *Beating Cancer with Nutrition*; Believes in beating cancer by strengthening the immune system via nutrition and he explains how he'd do it.
- Dr. Toni Bark: *Ketogenic Diet and Disease Reversal and Prevention* Alternative nutrition
- Jeffrey Smith IRT – *Concerned over GMOs (genetically modified organisms) and Cancer* – See online
- KC & Monica Craichy: *Discuss the importance of SuperFood Nutrition to Prevent Cancer* – Search online
- *"Budwig diet"*: https://www.cancertutor.com/budwig/ and other diets to strengthen immune system
- Mike Adams (LAB): *Heavy Metals and Cancer* – Via nutritional supplements, eating healthy, growing your own food – video: https://www.youtube.com/watch?v=_8cQVy6Zp0M
- Doug Kaufmann: *The Fungal Link to Cancer* - Asserts that *fungi* in foods may play a role in *cancer*. Sporanox – kills fungus – He says cancer is a fungus. Can it be killed using fungal myotoxin?

- Dr. David Jockers: *The Sugar-Cancer Connection* – The diet that destroys cancer.

Supplementation
I take the listed supplements, religiously. There may be days I feel my performance at the gym was sluggish without explanation until I realize I failed to take my morning or evening dosage of scheduled supplements.

Sleep
Good quality, uninterrupted sleep is a must to adequately recover and repair from my day's activities. Moreover, good, restful sleep is critical for cancer patients. I get over eight to nearly ten hours a night depending on the previous day's activities and how much I feel sapped. I refuse to deprive myself a good sleep. What's more, it reduces anxiety and stress.

When you try to go on less, it will eventually shorten your life. Men typically get up during the night to empty their bladder. The trick is to get right back to sleep. Don't look at the clock; it'll psych you into believing you've only x hours left before you get up, "anyways", so why not stay up? Don't fall into that self-made trap; ignore the clock!

Anxiety/ Stress Management
Some researchers believe there's a psychological/emotional link between high levels of anxiety/stress and all cancers. Negative emotion is one of the most toxically dangerous forms of oxidative stress known to cause physical damage to the human body. When this chemical state develops, cancer cells are better able to adapt and spread due to the patient's extreme stress levels.

Mismanaging your physical stress and emotional anxiety can genuinely put you in an early grave. I'm not perfect ... I've had a challenge recently that took away sleep time and thus temporarily lowered my immune system. I went into low intensity exercise, prayer and meditation which resulted in eventually getting the calming sleep I needed. And, afterwards? I prayed to give thanks.

In years past, I've been to therapy to get past emotionally difficult times (i.e., separation, divorce, breakups ...).To find coping skill sets that will work best, I've surfed the net, listened to cassettes, and read self-help material besides relying on therapy.

A solution is "out' there; it's up to you to find it. You're worth it!

For instance, take an online course, go to a half price bookstore, or take a class at night. If all else fails, it's wise and healthy to speak to a therapist. To effectively manage anxiety/stress, intervention may be necessary as in my case. It takes a strong man to recognize he needs help; your immune system will benefit when you make this choice, significantly.

Remember, too, to forgive all those who've offended you in years past and take it one step further. Ask God to "Please, bless them! For this practice to work, you have to genuinely "feel" the forgiveness and blessing. When this feeling is achieved, it has a powerful, lifting effect! I'm confident it will have a similar effect on you!

Like me, you're going to remember people you need to forgive and bless at the most inopportune times. Give yourself the necessary quiet time to completely release each person from their offense. It's God's way to ensure your anxiety/stress is effectively reduced as you're capable. Your immune system and recovery depends on it!

Exercise

To ensure adequate bone density, you have to be on some form of resistance/weight-bearing exercise program. The consequences when not engaging in exercise, regularly, are not pretty: instability; brittle bones; and you could end up in a wheelchair.

Now, I understand how different I am than most men. I began exercising as a teenager to improve performance in sports. What I found, though, was it was a great stress reliever which I desperately needed with all the dysfunction going on at home. As I got better at resistance exercise, I, quickly, became a successful competitor in three iron sports; Olympic weightlifting, power-lifting, and bodybuilding.

Aerobic exercise came later just before I turned 50. The health of my cardiovascular system was paramount if I was to successfully extend my life beyond the 70s. Although, my family did not have a history of heart issues, I was concerned about heart stroke and my resting heart rate. Thus, I began to use the treadmill/stationary bike as a means to get my rest heart rate below 70 to avoid heart issues. My research has found that after my initial 10 minute warm-up, 8-12 high intensity interval training (HIIT) works best for me.

I train five to six days a week about for 45-90 minutes each workout depending on what routine and body parts I'm training. I've one aerobic day, a core aerobic day, and 3-4 days of resistance exercise.

With regard to you and exercise, you're going to have to decide what's important in your life. Exercise can help you develop stronger cancer preventers/fighters in your system. What's more, your immune system will benefit, significantly, too.

A wonderful compliment paid to me is when people look up to me as their motivational driver. I'm their good example of what sound advice and good choices can achieve.

Hormonal Balance

I had no idea I was going to be impacted by a hormonal imbalance when I got my breast cancer. I'd heard women talk about hormones and believed men would be spared this predicament. How naive and ignorant to believe it was a notion and I'd never be affected! What compounded this belief was how rare anyone would hear that men were, also, affected by hormones.

I cannot emphasize the significance of hormonal balance between testosterone and estrogen/estradiol to minimize risks associated with disease including male breast cancer. When hormonal imbalance is determined, discuss with your PCP how balance can be returned. Begin getting checked for this balance/imbalance no later than age 50.

Since my MBC experience, I've been having my testosterone and estradiol checked nearly every quarter of every year without fail.

Lifestyle

The manner in which you manage yourself coupled with your habits; and how active/sedentary you are influences how healthy you will be as you age. In fact, the previously mentioned six characteristics are determined by your lifestyle choices. Remember, you are more likely to get any form of disease based on lifestyle choices than family history.

Noteworthy Comments

Although, I've spent much time researching mainstream treatments and natural healing alternatives, I wanted more validation. Was my choice to go natural in addition to formal treatment a good one? Thus, I've candidly discussed offline with several cancer medical professionals my findings. Here's what they said. Patients who choose other alternatives besides mainstream treatment were more likely to overcome/beat cancer than those who did not. Of course, it's always dependent on what stage the cancer was diagnosed, type of cancer, age, physical and emotional condition of the patient.

One last significant point, ensure your immune system is functioning at its best. See your PCP at least three times a year to monitor your health; take that annual Flu shot! Do whatever's necessary to maintain a robust immune system because without it, you potentially expose yourself to disease including cancer. Remember, those stem cells are waiting for a moment of weakness when recurrence is eminent.

Chapter
XIII
Wrap-up
and
Closing

Contradiction

Have you ever bragged that something's never happened to you and, then, it happens? My experience with cancer could not have been predicted. After all, I was invincible and men don't get breast cancer, remember?

Things change; I've done what I can to minimize additional recurrence. I wish "minimize" could be replaced with "prevent", but I'm a realist being an advanced age man. There's added risk brought on by my age. I'm controlling what I can to reduce the chance of having this invader enter my body, again. It's all going to depend on my immune system!

I fully realize I've active cancer stem cells inside me. According to mainstream information, they cannot be treated. On the other hand, other cancer professionals purport they know how to kill these stem cells, naturally.

Since my diagnosis July, 2012 and, then, again, in July, 2018, I've had indicators strongly suggesting I'm winning this battle. In spite, of having nine fewer lymph nodes to fight infection, reports say I've done exceptionally well. All chest, abdomen, pelvic area, and bone scans say it's been contained behind the chest wall since the beginning of this recurrence. Further, the University of Nebraska's study reinforced my belief that resistance training was significant for recovery. The naïve T-immune cells fight cancer and their presence might explain why my original tumor was pushing outward instead of attaching to my chest.

Did I suppose my brief use of steroids would have had a late effect on me more than a quarter of a century later? No! My ignorance about hormones and their balance was of no help, either. Going off steroids quickly than systemically reduced my natural production of testosterone. Imagine had I used longer what physical wreck I might've been in, today! My drive to compete and win against other steroid heads 30 some years ago became a prelude to what was in story for me at an advanced age.

It began when I failed to take my urologist's advice after this imbalance was discovered in my early 50s. Better disease management earlier in my life may have prevented what I had to face some years, later. Oh, I could lament over my mistakes, but, the outcome stays the same. So, take heed; reader, hormonal balance is significant in disease management and likely overlooked by too many.

The bottom line is chemical imbalance and age did me in regardless of my stellar lifestyle. I didn't have all the answers!

Adult male hormones start to change at about 30 years of age. Human growth hormone and testosterone production begins to falter while estrogen is on the rise. As you approach 50 and beyond, have your PCP include "T" and estradiol tests in your blood work to ensure these hormones are within an optimal 440-900ng/dL and 21-30pg/mL range, respectively. Note these ranges are not min-max, but optimal. When either hormone is out of range, begin therapy to make certain hormonal balance is restored.

My 2013 BRCA1 and BRCA2 gene blood tests indicated I had no gene mutations nor was I pre-programmed to acquire any cancers. Thus, I wouldn't be passing on any bad genes to my children. Nevertheless, I got breast cancer due to hormonal imbalance that lasted over a quarter century. Further, as I aged, that longstanding imbalance became significant. Too, I suspect my immune system was weakened by the imbalance and age which will never genuinely be known because they were never tested.

Recall my visit to MD Anderson's Integrated Medicine Center? I went there to determine how well I was eating and supplementing. Although, impressed with my exercise regimen, how well I ate, and what supplements I took, there was room for improvement. With few supplemental enhancements and several changes to my diet, I came out wiser. I had to smile, though, when the dietitian and doctor remarked they encouraged their patients to exercise at least once a week while I trained 5-6 days a week with regularity.

Based on my experience with MDA's Integrated Medicine Center, I advise you to meet with a professional dietitian to ensure your eating habits and supplementation adequately supports your overall health and lifestyle. Be mindful, part of acquiring cancer is derived from lifestyle choices. To live longer you may have to make significant change. Whatever your choice, all depends on how dear you hold life and how much longer you wish to live. Notwithstanding, quality of life is a serious consideration in your decision.

Lessons learned and new wisdom attained will always usher change. Most assuredly, I've made changes and with those changes I offer competent advice in hopes you'll make wiser choices before treatment. This value-added material should spare you some of the challenges I faced on my way to battle male breast cancer.

I can easily understand why some patients don't survive the treatment. Recovery can be aggravated by poor lifestyle choices throughout their life, a weakened immune system, and less than adequate physical condition. On top of that, you've the age factor. All depends on your physical condition and treatment tolerance. It's possible you could never experience many of the acute side effects during cancer treatment.

Ignorance, Again

I was clean of cancer until December, 2017 when it started all over, again with the flu. It weakened my immune system! My ignorance failed to see age had an effect on my immunity! I vow I'll never make that mistake, again and predict I'm fighting cancer for the last time! I expect no cancerous nodules will be found in this November's scan based on having applied natural healing alternatives learned earlier this year.

The Good

Although, things change, my integral core beliefs remained steadfast. Thank God for them! They've been significant in my personal battle with disease.

I'm told I've a zest for life and described as a man full of energy. I live life with purpose moving forward to conquer the next challenge. Nelson Mandella said it well, "I never lose! I either win or learn!" I've believed in those words way before I came across Mandella's quote. It simply validated what I had in myself!

The Not So Good

What I've gone through has been far from easy. It has taken away a physical part of me I've had all my life until surgery. I no longer have a left chest as I once knew it. Instead, there's a scar laced across the front of it to the underarm plus two puncture scars along my rib cage. There's no nipple or areola to balance what was once a man's chest. I've nine fewer lymph nodes which may or may not affect how my immune system will protect me in the future. I'll never be the same, again, and I'm reminded every single day of this disfigurement when I look in the mirror. If only I had the tumor checked/removed, sooner ...If only I took my doctor's advice in 2010, all this could have been avoided! If only ...If only!! I could go on beating myself up with what I didn't know. The good thing is you'll know better!

Although, I haven't experienced the emotional pain that a woman might face, I do know what it's like to not be physically the same ever again. That proclamation and reality is so irreversibly final. I'm forced to recognize it's a process of humility that may take the rest of my life or until I can capably reach some measure of acceptance. You see, I know too well what I've gone through is my entire fault!

Nearly every day I overthink how this entire encounter was brought on by my ignorance and failure to take my primary care physician's advice. The moment I knew it was benign, I insisted this tumor was inconsequential. I could treat it as I did when I was a teenager. It was going to go away. Little did I know this left alone benign tumor had a tenfold chance of converting to cancer. What angers me most is all I've gone through could have been avoided had wiser choices prevailed. Instead, my estrogen was given free rein for nearly one third of my life to chemically dominate my system as I aged. MBC was my consequence along with all the permanent side and late effects from treatment.

I fall back on how I'm more fortunate than many other MBC patients. My physical condition going in kept me from suffering many of the acute side effects. My preference for a more active, healthier lifestyle has produced a stronger immune system and helped me overcome the majority of most advanced age health issues. I don't take prescribed meds to manage my health; my liver doesn't have to work as hard. Even so, my physical condition and health standard wasn't enough to overcome all the treatment toxins and numerous permanently acquired aftereffects. I have not been completely exempt as you can attest from herein.

Interestingly, when I speak to medical professionals, I can sense they find me physically different. Often, I'm told I don't look, speak, behave, or dress like most men my age. Well, it's my lifestyle!

Frequently, when I meet new medical people, they usually start with, "What do you do?" as they critically look me over. So, I describe my background, health history as well as what activities I engage to stay fit. If need be, I tell them about my lifestyle, use of supplements, and eating regimen. As they grow at ease, conversation becomes more fluid.

Most medical people agree I'm not what they'd ordinarily expect. I just as a matter of factly explain "how I do it" with intense anaerobic and aerobic exercise, significant for me to maintain a healthy lifestyle and robust immune system. Where I see it as commonplace for me, they see it as exceptional.

In view of differences between the way I manage my life and most 80 something men, there haven't been studies to compare how different a fit body's system can respond to MDA's cancer treatment vs. the norm. What is normal?

For instance, I became critical of treatment conclusions. There's the question regarding fat and muscle fiber cells while undergoing chemo-therapy. My physical experience indicated chemo had in fact restricted/retarded the growth of all cells including fat and muscle fiber types. Researchers should take notice, except I surmise there're so few advanced aged athletes who've acquired any cancer type, they'd question the usefulness of their research time and effort. Why should it matter what affect treatment has on these few individuals? Except, it does matter to those who wish to continue maintaining their health and fitness under such extraordinary circumstances during treatment when fatigue and nausea permitted.

My beef!

What of the research, data, and statistics strictly focused on men? Since there're fewer than one percent (0.06%) of all annual breast cancer cases in the United States that are male, studies of men are typically merged with female breast cancer indicators. It's so inappropriate and discriminatory. Male chemistry is different than the female. Therefore, there should be independent studies strictly for men. However, it would mean change whose value would most likely be questioned by researchers.

Advisement

By the time you reach 50 and beyond if you've not been diagnosed with MBC, consider yourself fortunate. And if you have been diagnosed, my hope it was caught at an early stage.

Remember that managing your life to ensure health and longevity is ongoing. Begin, today. Maintain your vigilance with disease management considerations fully described, earlier.

By enlarge, you've control over your choices. You decide what you're willing to do to ensure a healthy immune system. As it gets stronger, you're likely to live a longer and healthier life.

In Review

Okay … Your biopsy/pathology report came back with the disheartening news; you've got male breast cancer!

There're significant steps you must work through to ensure you're informed as you can be before you move forward with a plan to beat this disease. Some of this information is review and worth repeating, here.

The moment you've been diagnosed, immediately, begin researching alternatives for treatment. Get treated as soon as is reasonable.

Ask questions; have the pathology report explained in an understandable manner. Knowing the stage and how aggressive the cancer is will determine the time you have to research treatment alternatives and minimize putting you at unnecessary risk. Know all the implications of your choices; permanent symptoms, side effects, and late effects

Relevant questions for your PCP and eventual cancer recovery team to answer:
- How did you get it
- What treatment alternatives are available
- Is the tumor fast or slow growing
- At what stage are you in
- How much time do you have to conduct your own research
- If the doctor you're speaking to or someone close to her/him was diagnosed with cancer, what treatment would they choose and why?
- When prescribed a drug as part of treatment, how likely will this drug cure you
- Is this or any prescribed drug on the American Cancer Society list as carcinogenic in humans
- If it is carcinogenic in humans, why has it been prescribed
- What're other complications of this drug
- What is the survivorship rate over a five year period for this treatment? Site the *Journal of Clinical Oncology* report, December, 2004
- What's the survivorship following treatment after five years?
- How will your cancer stem cells be treated?

Prior to treatment, there's the signing of agreement forms. Be certain all disclosures including potential permanent symptoms, side/late effects are revealed and discussed. Question where any doubt exists before anything is signed. If you're dissatisfied with the answers or not all questions could be answered, postpone signing until someone in authority can satisfy your queries.

Should you insist on chemo and radiation, remember the toxicities and warnings. Consider how chemo and radiation will permanently affect your body, health, and life.

Evaluate your physical condition to determine the potential outcome for you during and following treatment as well as five years and beyond.

Don't put all your trust in the hands of your medical team without questioning the methods of treatment.

Also, keep in mind according to mainstream recovery facilities, cancer stem cells still cannot be treated. They lay dormant inside you after treatment silently waiting for another opportune moment to create more cancer donor cells. To worsen matters, they'll be more aggressive the next time around. Whether cancer will surface a second time is dependent on your lifestyle choices and how well you've maintained your immune system following treatment.

Here's a serious consideration and contradiction. Either cancer stem cells can be killed utilizing Dr. Jockers' recommendations or they cannot be treated according to mainstream sources. I'd like to believe in Dr. Jockers' work, except where's the substantiated proof? Whatever you believe, maintaining a robust immune system to ward off disease including cancer is a must! Choice may once more determine if sickness will disrupt your life, again.

My Message to You

Different people handle matters like this one, differently. Remember, I was scared after my diagnosis and the start of treatment in 2012. One major lesson I learned was I couldn't control what was happening to me. I had to learn to stop beating myself up; find a way to release the emotional pain and fear. I turned it over to my Higher Power, but, I kept taking "it" back. Expect it will happen to you, too.

Life and mortality can be a bitch. I've learned much throughout my life that crystallized before me and was revalidated that fateful day in July, 2012. I had to talk and be with those I cared about/who cared about me in my family as well as stay close with friends. I grew weary of facing my reality and vowed I wouldn't be a victim. I wanted some control over what "things" were destined to happen to me during this period. My drive to research MBC and write about it became a healthy diversion and, actually, got me past the scary stuff. Staying active in the gym during my treatment (when nausea and fatigue allowed) was another constructive distraction for me.

I encourage you to stay the course, find diversions/distractions, besides what you'd ordinarily do every day.

Yes, it's tough grappling with a diagnosis. I'm genuinely sorry it has come this far. Nobody really knows what to say without offending or saying something that could be interpreted as negative. I hated hearing *"It's going to be okay …"* People meant well with this well-intended knee-jerk response, but it tore my insides apart whenever I heard it! I'd break eye contact from the well-wisher and think, *"There's no way in friggin' hell that anyone would know everything's going to be alright."*

On a personal note, I wish this wasn't happening to you and the news must have been devastating for you to share with those you care about. Just know your loved ones are there for you and thinking about you! My hope is you're holding up well under these challenging circumstances. During my time of duress, I was reminded that "… this too shall pass …"

A Closing Thought
Have you ever wondered what this growth looked like after its removal from your chest? Of course, the size will vary depending on how much time you took before diagnosis.

Picture being on a sunny, sandy beach; it's a pleasant day, not too hot, not too cool. You can see the pale beige colored sand for miles to your left and right as you approach the shoreline, barefoot. The loose, warm sand massages your feet with each step. A soft breeze catches your hair as you bend down to wet your hands. Pick up a small bit of sand to pack like you would a small-sized mound. Make it more conical and irregular; it shouldn't be larger than an inch at the base and no taller than a half inch. Let the dampness of the water bind to the sand; pack it well into that odd, tapering shape. Notice how the sunlight causes some of the crystalline mass to glitter like damp sand would. Now, change that beige color to a light gray with bits of white and pale red throughout.

Look at it for a while and remember a tumor similar to that mass was in your chest behind your nipple. It was growing and growing ever so slowly until you decided to have it diagnosed and removed.

Imagine how much more trouble you'd have if that ugly, gritty mass had grown larger and its cancer cells spread throughout your body. Think about it; … you were lucky, weren't you?

Now, spread the word … men can get this cancer, you know the signs; talk about it. Let people know it's no joke!!

In the Interim

If you've questions, I may have answers. Please, write me at
bovairdbusiness@wt.net
Populate the subject line to avoid your email from rolling over to my Spam file. Thank you.

Remember, you'll have a better time managing yourself and your cancer due to the material in this book.

God Bless you!

Made in the USA
Columbia, SC
09 October 2020